100 Questions & Answers About Your High-Risk Pregnancy

DEC   2008

Elizabeth S. Platt
Buxton, Maine

Michael G. Pinette, MD
Division of Maternal-Fetal Medicine
Maine Medical Center
Portland, Maine

Betty Campbell, RN
Division of Maternal-Fetal Medicine
Maine Medical Center
Portland, Maine

Andrea Tetreau, RN
Division of Maternal-Fetal Medicine
Maine Medical Center
Portland, Maine

JONES AND BARTLETT PUBLISHERS
Sudbury, Massachusetts
BOSTON   TORONTO   LONDON   SINGAPORE

World Headquarters
Jones and Bartlett Publishers
40 Tall Pine Drive
Sudbury, MA 01776
978-443-5000
info@jbpub.com
www.jbpub.com

Jones and Bartlett Publishers
Canada
6339 Ormindale Way
Mississauga, Ontario L5V 1J2
CANADA

Jones and Bartlett Publishers
International
Barb House, Barb Mews
London W6 7PA
UK

Jones and Bartlett's books and products are available through most bookstores and online booksellers. To contact Jones and Bartlett Publishers directly, call 800-832-0034, fax 978-443-8000, or visit our Web Site, www.jbpub.com.

Substantial discounts on bulk quantities of Jones and Bartlett's publications are available to corporations, professional associations, and other qualified organizations. For details and specific discount information, contact the special sales department at Jones and Bartlett via the above contact information or send an email to specialsales@jbpub.com.

The authors, editor, and publisher have made every effort to provide accurate information. However, they are not responsible for errors, omissions, or for any outcomes related to the use of the contents of this book and take no responsibility for the use of the products and procedures described. Treatments and side effects described in this book may not be applicable to all people; likewise, some people may require a dose or experience a side effect that is not described herein. Drugs and medical devices are discussed that may have limited availability controlled by the Food and Drug Administration (FDA) for use only in a research study or clinical trial. Research, clinical practice, and government regulations often change the accepted standard in this field. When consideration is being given to use of any drug in the clinical setting, the health care provider or reader is responsible for determining FDA status of the drug, reading the package insert, and reviewing prescribing information for the most up-to-date recommendations on dose, precautions, and contraindications, and determining the appropriate usage for the product. This is especially important in the case of drugs that are new or seldom used.

The authors, editor and publisher of this publication have reviewed and accepted editorial changes provided by sanofi-aventis, Inc.

Production Credits
Executive Publisher: Christopher Davis
Associate Editor: Kathy Richardson
Production Editor: Rachel Rossi
Editorial Assistant: Jessica Acox
Associate Marketing Manager: Ilana Goddess

Manufacturing Buyer: Therese Connell
Composition: Appingo Publishing Services
Cover Design: Kristin E. Ohlin
Printing and Binding: Malloy, Inc.
Cover Printing: Malloy, Inc.

Library of Congress Cataloging-in-Publication Data

Platt, Elizabeth.
  100 questions & answers about your high-risk pregnancy / Elizabeth S. Platt.
    p. cm.
  ISBN-13: 978-0-7637-5573-7
  ISBN-10: 0-7637-5573-7
  1. Pregnancy--Complications--Miscellanea. 2. Labor (Obstetrics)--Complications--Miscellanea.
I. Title. II. Title: One hundred questions and answers about your high-risk pregnancy.
  RG571.P63 2008
  618.2--dc22

                         2008022641
6048
Printed in the United States of America
12 11 10 09 08   10 9 8 7 6 5 4 3 2 1

618.2
8

For Amy, with hope, and for Nathaniel and Eric,
who are worth every minute of it.

CONTENTS

Questions 1–8 provide background on what constitutes a high-risk pregnancy, including:
- What happens during a normal pregnancy?
- What problems can occur in pregnancy?
- Why is my pregnancy considered high risk?

Questions 9–16 address concerns about the tests that parents can undertake to determine potential problems with a high-risk pregnancy, such as:
- What is prenatal testing? When are more specialized prenatal tests needed?
- What are the benefits of prenatal testing? Will testing help reduce my risk of problems in pregnancy?
- What prenatal tests are available? What do they show?

Questions 16–32 discuss how preexisting health factors in the mother can affect pregnancy, including:
- Why am I considered to be "high risk" just because I'm over 35? How does my age affect my risk for complications?
- I do a lot of running and sports, and my doctor told me I should cut back on some of my activities. Why? Isn't exercise good during pregnancy?
- Why does my doctor think that I may be at risk for preterm labor or other complications?

I first came up with the concept for this book as something of a joke. In 2004, I had been working on Jones and Bartlett's *100 Questions & Answers* series for almost two years. When I was having difficulty getting pregnant, I griped to Chris Davis, the medical publisher at Jones and Bartlett and a long-time colleague, that I would soon be writing *100 Questions & Answers About Infertility* but, happily, was soon able to announce that I'd changed the title of my next book to *100 Questions & Answers About Your High-Risk Pregnancy*. He didn't get the joke at first, but then, neither one of us knew that the joke was really on me. Although my off-the-cuff remark was referring specifically to my age (I was 38), I had no way of knowing that a number of complications lay ahead, including a partial placenta previa and pregnancy-induced hypertension and preeclampsia that put me on bed rest for a month. Even at the end, stalled labor turned childbirth into a 33-hour marathon overshadowed by uncertainty. Was the baby okay? Would I have the strength to push when the time came? Would I need a C-section?

In the end, however, everything turned out just fine. My son Nathaniel came through with flying colors. I had the strength when I needed it (with a little help from the anesthesiologist), and no cesarean was required. Nathaniel, now 3 years old, is a healthy, happy little boy, and I'm in excellent health and enjoying parenthood.

I want to accomplish one particular thing with this book: Reassurance that *risk* and *probability* are not the same as inevitable and that complications are not necessarily life-and-death struggles, although this perspective is hard to keep while dealing with problems. This message is essential for anyone facing a high-risk pregnancy—as I did, again, having found out four days before starting the book that my (unexpected) second child was on his way. Although my past history of complications made me worry that I'd experience similar problems, as it turned out, there was only one—a relatively minor complication completely unrelated to any of my prior problems—and it was resolved very early on; the rest of the pregnancy was relatively uneventful. My younger son, Eric, 10 months old as I write this, is healthy and strong after a blessedly mundane pregnancy, labor, and delivery. The second pregnancy was considerably less difficult, in part because I had much more information and because I had experienced complications and thus knew that they can be, and usually are, successfully resolved.

It isn't exactly news that more women are having their first children later in their lives, nor is it shocking to hear stories of "miracle babies" who are born to supposedly infertile women with the assistance of modern medicine; indeed, current controversy now centers around *how old is too old*, as women in their late 40s, 50s, and even 60s are having babies with the help of modern fertility methods. You don't often hear of these advances in obstetrical medicine in terms of an increase in high-risk pregnancy; nevertheless, that's exactly what has been going on: In the past 20 or 30 years, the rate of pregnancies being categorized as high risk has skyrocketed.

"High-risk pregnancy" has such an ominous sound that women when hearing it may feel anxious and spend a great deal of time worrying that something will go wrong when they *should* be feeling joyful expectation (sandwiched around the bouts of hormones, nausea, swollen feet, aching back, and other less pleasant symptoms that go along with the entire process). Realistically, there's *always* a chance of something going wrong, whether your pregnancy is high risk or not—in the greater scheme of things, however, even with high-risk situations, the chances that a problem will occur are considerably less than the odds of having a normal, problem-free pregnancy that ends with a healthy baby and a happy (if tired) mother.

All of the authors have seen frightening situations that turned out successfully. At Maine Medical Center, the Maternal-Fetal Medicine division treats, as Dr. Pinette puts it, the "sickest of the sickest": Women who have had organ transplants, severe cardiovascular disease, cancer, and other seemingly insurmountable health problems have gone on to bear healthy babies. Many of these women had been told by other doctors to simply forget the idea of having a child—and most of them probably faced more severe complications than the problems that have caused you to open this book. So take heart! You are not alone, and others in similar (and worse) situations to yours have come through to a happy ending.

Elizabeth Platt
Michael Pinette, MD
Betty Campbell, RN
Andrea Tetreau, RN

ACKNOWLEDGMENTS

In both my pregnancies, I had excellent care from a collection of smart, knowledgeable people. I thank the staff at The Women's Health Clinic of Cambridge Hospital in Cambridge, Massachusetts, particularly Kate Harney, MD, who saw me through every anxious step of my first pregnancy and referred me to Maine Medical Center when problems began in my second. Special thanks are given to "Quick Rick" in the Cambridge Hospital delivery room for a memorably fast and effective epidural when I was almost at the end of my rope. Likewise, I thank the staff of the Maternal-Fetal Medicine Division at the Maine Medical Center in Portland, Maine, particularly those directly involved in my care: Michael Pinette, MD, Joseph Wax, MD, John Pulvino, MD, Betty Campbell, RN, Andrea Tetreau, RN, and Jennifer Falk, RN. Thanks also to everyone at Jones and Bartlett Publishers, Inc., especially Chris Davis, Anne Spencer, Rachel Rossi, and the entire production department; your support through both pregnancies (and their aftermaths) was an essential ingredient to their success. I could not have survived either motherhood or book writing without the support of my family and friends: my mother, Nancy Van Dyke Platt, my stepdaughter Marcayla Hamblin, my "personal trainer" Sharyn Rose, Karen Ferreira, Stephanie Bunn, Nina Ghareeb, Shellie Newell, Debbie Rebelo, and the various other people who kept me going when things were dicey. Thanks also to Amy O'Keefe for her valuable comments on the manuscript. Finally, a huge debt of gratitude is owed to my partner, birth coach, baby daddy, best friend, and significant source of irritation (sometimes), Mark Hamblin. Thanks for doing your best to avoid all the potholes en route to the hospital, and sorry about the squashed fingers.

Elizabeth Platt

PART ONE

The Basics

What happens during a normal pregnancy?

What problems can occur in pregnancy?

Why is my pregnancy considered high risk?

More . . .

Fetus

Developmental stage during pregnancy occurring after about 8 weeks of the pregnancy until birth.

Risk

A determination of the probability of a particular event that takes into account specific contributing factors.

Probability

A measurement of the likelihood of an event actually occurring.

1. What happens during a normal pregnancy?

An entire book can be written about normal pregnancy, and indeed, you've probably already bought one (or several). Most of these describe at length the changes in the growing **fetus** and focus on the types of symptoms that are typical in pregnancy; nevertheless, some of the significant physiological events within a *normal* pregnancy need to be distinguished from those problems that cause you to be considered *high risk*.

WHAT IS RISK?

Before we get into the nitty-gritty details of normal pregnancy, let's take a moment to define the most important term that we'll use in this book: **risk**. Risk is a measurement of **probability**—the likelihood of an event (generally unwelcome) occurring—in a particular set of circumstances, taking into account all known contributing factors. In pregnancy, the events that cause concern are those situations in the mother, the baby, or both that could lead to serious health problems or death for one or both during the pregnancy, at birth, or shortly after birth.

Most people don't keep risk and probability in proper perspective—understandably, as here we're talking about potential problems with one's unborn child(ren), a matter of extreme concern to would-be parents. Probability measurements are a squishy, gray area in which something isn't necessarily black or white, positive or negative. They are estimates, not certainties, which is particularly hard on mothers and fathers who, having been told of a possible risk, want to know *for certain* whether they need to be concerned that this problem will occur. Being given a probability instead of a certainty is frustrating and can be frightening, but to effectively cope with risk, you must understand what those odds are and what they mean. Then you must set the goal of doing everything possible to beat the odds and have a good result.

When patients come in for their first appointment, we like to give them the following example of what constitutes risk. Nearly all of our patients travel by car to our offices in Portland. This entails a certain amount of risk of getting into an accident. The risk of an accident, however, increases or decreases depending on a number of factors: the time of day, the weather, how far you're driving, how fast you drive, whether your car is well maintained, and many others. You could have one or several factors at play on any given occasion, but even people traveling at high speeds for 50 miles during rush hour in rain and snow in a beat-up old sedan make it safely to their destinations *most of the time*, far more often than not. Thus, factors that increase your risk of an accident don't necessarily mean that you won't arrive safely. The same is true of pregnancy: Many factors could potentially increase your risk of having a problem, but most of the time you'll still end up with a healthy baby.

Any number of pregnancy complications might occur, and some of them are extremely worrisome. It is extremely important that you understand one thing when you and your doctor discuss the risk of a complication or a poor outcome: *Being at risk, even high risk, does not mean that you are 100% certain to have a problem occur*, nor does it automatically mean that you'll have a bad outcome even if complications *do* arise. This may sound like a cliché, but a positive frame of mind can be your best strategy in avoiding complications, as well as in improving the final result if complications arise. The reality is that most maternal complications, even severe ones, can be managed successfully.

Most maternal complications, even severe ones, can be managed successfully.

NORMAL PREGNANCY

Now back to our original subject: what happens during normal pregnancy. The main difference between what you will read here and what you might read elsewhere is that we'll describe what happens in the mother's body, where most pregnancy books will talk about the baby's growth and focus

Ovaries

Reproductive organs in women where eggs (ova) are stored and certain hormones are released.

Ovulates

The release of an egg in the ovaries midway through a woman's reproductive cycle.

Ovum

Egg.

Fallopian tube

Tube connecting the ovaries to the uterus, through which an egg passes after ovulation.

Sperm

Male reproductive cell that joins with an ovum to initiate pregnancy.

Blastocyst

Early stage of a fertilized egg in which the egg divides and forms a hollow ball before implantation in the uterus.

Placenta

Specialized organ that develops to supply oxygen and nutrients to a growing fetus.

only a little on the physical changes in the mother. Why do it this way? Because risk factors affecting *only* the baby are relatively uncommon, while risk factors affecting the mother (or the mother and baby together) are fairly common.

FIRST TRIMESTER

As you're probably aware, the female reproductive tract consists principally of the **ovaries**, fallopian tubes, uterus, cervix, and vagina (see Figure 1). A normal pregnancy begins when a woman **ovulates**, releasing a single **ovum** ("egg") that travels down into her **fallopian tube**. If she has had sexual intercourse within 3 to 5 days preceding this event, or even a short time

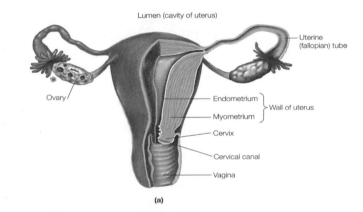

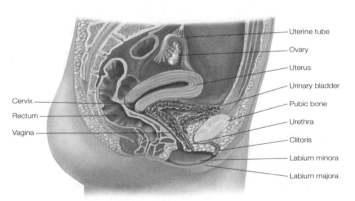

Figure 1   Anatomy of the female reproductive tract. (A) Frontal view. (B) Side view.
SOURCE: Chiras, *Human Biology, 6th Edition*, 2008: Jones and Bartlett Publishers LLC, Sudbury, MA. www.jbpub.com. Reprinted with permission.

afterward, then somewhere within the fallopian tube the egg meets the **sperm** and is fertilized. It begins to divide and to form a hollow ball of cells. This ball of cells is called a **blasto-cyst** (Figure 2); its outer portion will eventually become the **placenta** while the inner portion develops into the **embryo**. The blastocyst continues to travel down the fallopian tube into the uterus, taking about 4 days. It floats freely in the **uterus** for about 3 to 5 more days, sustained by secretions of the uterine lining, before implanting within the uterine wall at about the 9th or 10th day (Figure 3). At this point, the placental cells begin producing a hormone called **human chorionic gonado-trophin (hCG)**, which stops the ovaries from producing more eggs and signals the ovaries to produce more **progesterone**, a hormone that prevents the woman from having a period. At the same time, these cells begin to develop into the placenta, a temporary organ connecting the uterine wall with the embryo via the **umbilical cord**.

The Basics

Embryo

Developmental stage during pregnancy occurring after implantation in the uterus and before about 8 weeks of the pregnancy.

Uterus

Female reproductive organ used for carrying the fetus during pregnancy.

Human chorionic gonadotrophin (hCG)

A hormone produced by the placenta that prevents menstruation and ovulation.

Progesterone

A female hormone with several important roles in pregnancy.

Umbilical cord

The cord connecting the placenta to the fetus.

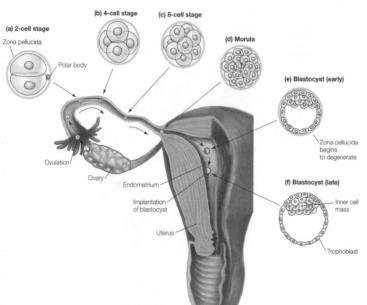

Figure 2   Formulation of the morula and blastocyst during pre-embryonic development.
SOURCE: Chiras, *Human Biology, 5th Edition*, 2005: Jones and Bartlett Publishers LLC, Sudbury, MA. www.jbpub.com. Reprinted with permission.

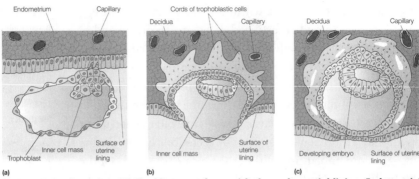

(a) (b) (c)

Figure 3 Implantation. (A) The blastocyst fuses with the endometrial lining. Endometrial cells proliferate, forming the decidua. (B) The blastocyst digests its way into the endometrium. Cords of trophoblastic cells invade, digesting maternal tissue and providing nutrients for the developing blastocyst. (C) The blastocyst soon becomes completely embedded in the endometrium.

SOURCE: Chiras, *Human Biology, 5th Edition*, 2005: Jones and Bartlett Publishers LLC, Sudbury, MA. www.jbpub.com. Reprinted with permission.

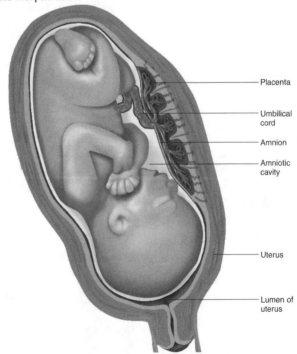

Figure 4 The placenta. This organ, made from maternal and fetal tissue, helps nourish the developing fetus and remove wastes. It also produces important hormones.

SOURCE: Chiras, *Human Biology, 5th Edition*, 2005: Jones and Bartlett Publishers LLC, Sudbury, MA. www.jbpub.com. Reprinted with permission.

The placenta has two specific functions: (1) transferring nutrients and oxygen from the mother's blood into that of the embryo and (2) filtering waste and carbon dioxide from the embryo to be eliminated by the mother. Its development into a fully functional organ spans the full 12 weeks of the first trimester, but it begins to serve its intended purpose almost immediately (Figure 4).

When do we use the terms *embryo* versus *fetus* versus *baby*?

In medicine, an embryo is the earliest stage of development after the fertilized egg has become embedded in the uterus, lasting from week 1 to week 8. It is referred to as a fetus only after it has developed to a point of being recognizably human—usually at about 8 weeks. Before that time, if you were to compare it with the embryo of a dog, cat, or other mammal, you wouldn't be able to detect much difference in their appearance; by 8 weeks, however, the characteristics that distinguish a human from any other animal are generally present. The early fetal stage occurs between 8 and 13 weeks, and at this point, maternal/fetal specialists are able to distinguish signs of normal (or abnormal) development. After birth, we refer to the fetus as a **newborn** or **neonate** (from the Latin neo = new and natus = born).

The term "baby" isn't a medical term—it's a parental term. It's a term of anticipation, hope, and excitement and sometimes a bit of nervousness or even dread. For an expectant parent, an embryo is a baby, a fetus is a baby, and a newborn is also a baby—the term describes a relationship, not a biological category. In this book, which is intended to be read by expectant parents, we use *baby* interchangeably with *embryo*, *fetus*, and *newborn* if we're not discussing specific biological characteristics of the stage of development.

During these early weeks, the mother experiences the first physical changes related to pregnancy—breast soreness, lack of menstrual periods, fatigue, and more frequent urination. Table 1 gives a summary of the physical changes that a pregnant woman undergoes throughout the course of pregnancy—and it's easy to see that the effects are considerable! Not all changes happen right away, however, nor do all of them last throughout the pregnancy. Everyone's favorite symptom, morning sickness—more accurately called **nausea and vomiting of pregnancy**, as it doesn't always occur in the morning—usually

The Basics

Newborn/neonate

A newly born infant; a baby less than a month old.

Nausea and vomiting of pregnancy

A symptom of pregnancy commonly occurring in the first trimester.

Table 1 Physical Changes and Symptoms Experienced by a Pregnant Woman During a Normal Pregnancy

Body system	Changes	Symptoms
Endocrine (hormones)	Production of hormones by pituitary, thyroid, parathyroid, and adrenal glands increases, in some cases dramatically. The placenta develops into an additional endocrine organ.	Nearly all pregnancy-related symptoms are related to these endocrine changes. Mood swings, food cravings or aversions, fatigue, and sleeplessness may all stem from hormonal changes.
Cardiovascular (heart and blood vessels)	Total volume of blood in the body increases 30–50%. Blood vessels become dilated due to higher progesterone levels, so blood pressure falls, reaching its lowest point during the second trimester. White blood cell count increases substantially, but red cells increase at a somewhat slower pace.	Increased heart rate; puffiness in fingers, ankles; dizziness or faintness; fatigue.
Gastrointestinal (stomach and intestines)	Increased hCG levels in early pregnancy affects gastric system. Smooth muscles of stomach and intestines relax due to high progesterone levels. Expanding uterus places pressure on blood vessels in the lower pelvic region.	Nausea and vomiting, sometimes severe, from about week 6 onward; heartburn, constipation, and other discomfort; hemorrhoids.
Respiratory (lungs)	Lungs adjust to provide increased amounts of oxygen to meet the needs of both mother and fetus. Pressure on the lungs by the growing uterus is offset by flaring of the rib cage to allow the lungs to expand sideways. Oxygen consumption increases by 20%, and respiratory rate increases by 1 to 2 breaths per minute.	Shortness of breath, especially in later weeks of pregnancy; dizziness or faintness.

Body system	Changes	Symptoms
Reproductive (uterus, birth canal, breasts)	Uterus expands to 20 times its original size to accommodate the fetus as it grows. Higher estrogen levels cause the cervix to soften and produce more mucus, which plugs the cervical opening until labor begins. Elevated estrogen and progesterone halt egg production in the ovaries. Estrogen also prepares the birth canal by promoting increased vascularity in the vagina, thickening of the mucous membranes, and loosening ligaments in the pelvis. Breasts increase in size and fatty composition in preparation for milk production; colostrum is produced by the 16th week of pregnancy.	Breast tenderness, increased size of breasts, thickened vaginal discharge, colostrum dripping from nipples; menstrual periods usually cease but some women experience spotting.
Musculoskeletal (bones, muscles, tendons, and ligaments)	Relaxin and progesterone cause ligaments and joints to soften and loosen in preparation for birth. Changes in posture due to uterine growth occur. Muscles in the abdominal wall sometimes separate.	Back pain, pressure and discomfort in the pelvis and legs; shooting pains down the left leg (sciatica); poor balance; vertigo; increased susceptibility to injury, particularly joint or tendon injuries.
Integumentary (skin)	Pigmentation and texture of the skin changes due to hormones and stretching as uterus and breasts increase in size. Skin problems such as acne or psoriasis may increase or may disappear altogether.	Stretch marks, acne, itching, darkening of areola, dark line on belly, dark "mask" on face. Hair is often noticeably thicker and nails grow faster.
Other	Changes in vision as increase in body fluids affects the shape of the retina; increase in body temperature; increased sense of smell coupled with intolerance to strong odors.	Blurred vision, discomfort wearing contact lenses; a feeling of being feverish.

Areola

The circle of dark, sensitive skin surrounding the nipple of each breast.

Hormones

Chemicals produced by various organs to produce specific responses by body systems.

Estrogen

A female reproductive hormone.

Estriol

A variant of estrogen that is produced primarily by the placenta during pregnancy.

Thyroxine

A hormone produced by the thyroid gland.

Prostaglandin

A hormone-like substance important in the contraction and relaxation of smooth muscle, the dilation and constriction of blood vessels, control of blood pressure, and modulation of inflammation.

Prolactin

A hormone that is associated with milk production.

begins around the sixth week but can start earlier, later, or not at all. The mother's body temperature often rises noticeably, making her feel as if she has a slight fever; she also may feel bloated, as her body has begun to produce additional fluids. These excess fluids may show up as a stuffy nose, drippy sinuses, and sometimes even drooling. The mother's heart and kidneys are working a great deal harder to support the developing fetus, and this is reflected in her increased heart rate (by anywhere from 10 to 20 beats per minute), elevated blood pressure, and frequent urination. Skin changes, particularly darkening of the **areola** of the breast and, occasionally, dark patches on the face and abdomen (called melasma) sometimes occur during this phase. Mood swings, weepiness, and stress are also common during the first trimester.

The cause of these symptoms is primarily the hormonal changes that accompany pregnancy. **Hormones** are chemicals that are produced by various organs; they act as messengers to instruct the body's systems to respond in specific ways to specific physiological situations. Pregnancy is one such situation; it inspires massive release of a number of different hormones from the reproductive organs, the thyroid, pituitary, and adrenal glands, certain sectors of the brain, and—it may surprise you to learn—from the placenta and the fetus itself. Various forms of **estrogen**, particularly a variant called **estriol**, which comes mainly from the placenta, increase dramatically in early pregnancy, as do progesterone, hCG, and **thyroxine** (thyroid hormone). In the case of some of these, specifically hCG and thyroxine, the increase is temporary—the hormones support embryonic/fetal development to a point and then decline when they are no longer needed. Other hormones and hormone-like chemicals, including **prostaglandin, prolactin, oxytocin,** and **human placental lactogen (HPL)**, are present in smaller amounts at the early stages but gradually increase and reach peak levels near the end of the pregnancy. These hormones have a greater impact on labor, delivery, and milk production than on the maintenance of pregnancy; therefore, they aren't required in large amounts until the pregnancy nears term.

Most symptoms in the first trimester are side effects of the hormonal increase—some that serve a useful purpose (the increase in body fluids, although uncomfortable for the mother, ensures that the fetus has sufficient nutrition, waste removal, and oxygen to survive and grow) and others that serve no significant purpose and are downright annoying (color changes to the skin, for example). Some symptoms, however, are related to purely physical changes. Changes in the size and shape of the uterus, for example, cause it to press on the bladder, causing the mother to urinate more frequently. Weight gain and uterine growth may also throw off the mother's center of balance, adding to fatigue, dizziness, and even nausea as she tries to compensate for the changes.

Unfortunately, it is difficult to know when these symptoms are simply standard pregnancy-related discomfort and when they're an outward sign of a real problem. Every pregnancy is different, and some fairly serious disorders have symptoms that are identical to common, garden-variety pregnancy complaints. For this reason, most physicians request that routine tests are performed after pregnancy has been confirmed. These tests obtain **baseline** information on the mother's physical condition and screen for common problems so that they can be treated (and hopefully resolved) before significant harm occurs to either the mother or the developing fetus. Some of these tests take place between the 8th and 13th week; others must wait until later stages of fetal development.

The earliest routine tests usually include the following:

- Blood tests are given to determine blood type and **Rh status** (that is, whether your blood type is "positive" or "negative," as well as whether antibodies have developed against your baby's Rh type; see Question 33), to check levels of hormones such as hCG and thyroxine (which can provide clues to problems in the functioning of the placenta or the thyroid gland), and to obtain a **complete blood count (CBC)**. The CBC checks the status of all

---

Oxytocin

A hormone and neurotransmitter that is important in labor.

Human placental lactogen (HPL)

A hormone produced by the placenta that interferes with insulin to promote growth in the fetus.

The Basics

Baseline

The starting point; in medicine, the normal values for a given person.

Rh status

The presence or absence of a specific blood factor that can determine the risk of hemolytic disease of the newborn.

Complete blood count (CBC)

An analysis of the various blood cells to determine whether any blood-related health issues are present.

Anemia
Low red blood cell count.

Thrombocytopenia
Low platelet count.

Leukemia
Any of several forms of cancer affecting the white blood cells.

of the major blood cells to make sure that the mother doesn't have preexisting blood disorders such as **anemia** (insufficient or ineffective red blood cells), **thrombocytopenia** (low platelets), infections, **leukemia**, or any other disorders affecting white blood cells. Aside from anemia, which is relatively common, most of these diseases and disorders are unusual, but detecting them early can be an important factor in preventing complications in the pregnancy.

• Other tests, either blood tests or skin tests, check to see whether the mother has antibodies that are specific to infectious diseases that can affect pregnancy. The tests that are performed as a routine matter vary depending on the laws of each state and/or hospital policies. Some diseases, such as chickenpox, rubella, hepatitis B, tuberculosis, cytomegalovirus, syphilis, gonorrhea, and chlamydia are generally included in routine testing so that the infection, if present, can be treated immediately to prevent any effects on the fetus. Testing for some other diseases, particularly HIV, may be offered to the mother but are included only if she consents to the test.

• Depending on your family history and ethnicity, genetic tests are performed to screen for fetal abnormalities such as cystic fibrosis, sickle cell anemia, Tay-Sachs, thalassemia, or other genetic diseases. Cystic fibrosis, for example, is particularly common among Caucasians, while sickle-cell anemia is common in people of African descent, and Tay-Sachs is mainly found in people descended from Eastern European Jews.

• Urinalysis to screen for protein, sugar, white blood cells, blood, and bacteria in the urine may offer clues about undetected infections or underlying diseases that may have few symptoms. Kidney or bladder disorders, pregnancy-induced hypertension, and urinary tract infections can be detected through urine tests. Urine checks are a routine part of all obstetrical visits, particularly for the mother who might be at risk for hypertension or kidney disease.

- Heartbeat monitoring with a handheld Doppler device may be done near the end of the first trimester, usually at about 12 weeks. Although the baby's heartbeat can sometimes be heard as early as 10 weeks, most practitioners will wait until at least 12 weeks to begin using the Doppler simply because it's considerably easier to pick up the heartbeat on the device. Although handheld Doppler devices are becoming readily available, they should be used with caution. The fact that anyone *can* use them doesn't mean anyone *should* use them. A Doppler device actually puts out more energy than an ultrasound, so it's not necessarily safe to use it for fetal monitoring on a regular (daily) basis unless there is cause for significant concern. So if you had visions of buying one to keep tabs on your baby, you should understand that it's not a very good idea. Just remember, our grandmothers didn't have the opportunity to listen to the baby's heartbeat either, and they managed just fine!
- At about week 28, an oral glucose tolerance test is used to check for signs of gestational diabetes (see Question 52).
- The use of ultrasound evaluation is becoming routine in the first trimester, but at this stage, the **ultrasound specialist** can't really see much of the fetus's internal structure—its organs, bones, and so forth—so any problems or abnormalities that exist will often not be detectable (although highly experienced centers can sometimes detect major birth defects at the end of the first trimester). If a pregnancy is clearly established, the woman's menstrual history is well known, and there are no obvious "red flags," such as bleeding or cramping, the obstetrician may wait until the fetus is more developed before calling for an ultrasound evaluation of the fetus. An ultrasound, however, *can* be used to establish the gestational age of the fetus if the mother's menstrual cycles were irregular or absent. It has also become fairly common to use ultrasound as part of a **first trimester screening**, which combines ultrasound with specific

Ultrasound specialist

A medical professional trained in the use of ultrasound scanning to assess and diagnose pregnancy and pregnancy-related disorders.

First trimester screening

A combination of blood and urine tests and ultrasound screening to look for early signs of complications in the first trimester.

The Basics

blood tests to determine whether there is a need to undergo more advanced prenatal tests for chromosomal abnormalities (see Questions 9–14). The use of ultrasound for this purpose is called a **nuchal translucency scan**; it is performed between weeks 11 and 14 of the pregnancy, as further described in Question 14.

Nuchal translucency scan

An ultrasound analysis in the first trimester used to assess the risk of certain congenital disorders, especially Down syndrome.

Screening tests

Diagnostic tools used to assess a risk of specific disorders in pregnancy.

Nearly all of these tests are **screening tests**; that is, they look for results that are outside of the generally accepted normal range for an average pregnant woman. They do not provide definitive yes or no answers about whether a problem does or does not exist—they simply provide estimates of a woman's risk level. Sometimes, a perfectly normal, healthy baby in a healthy, average mother will produce suspicious test results for unknown reasons; alternatively, it's also quite possible that a health complication in a mother or a fetus will go undetected because the test results are within normal parameters. Like most tools, these tests are only as good as the person who uses them; thus, more accurate detection of problems is likely when the tests are performed by experienced staff.

A Note About Ultrasounds

You should know two important facts about ultrasound. First, many concerns (and myths) exist regarding the safety of ultrasound. Current evidence indicates that an ultrasound performed at an accredited facility is safe. Accreditation is based on standards set by the American College of Radiology and/or the American Institute of Ultrasound in Medicine for how the machinery is used and calibrated. Your hospital or ultrasound facility should have a notice of accreditation for you to see. Second, seeing the fetus in an ultrasound image is one of the first occasions that parents bond with their infant. **Ultrasound bonding**, as we call it, is a mixed bag because although it increases the parents' sense of connectedness to their child, that bond also increases the stress and anxiety if the pregnancy has complications—to put it simply, the parents care and worry more about a child made visible to them by ultrasound. This minor drawback of ultrasound bonding is far outweighed by its benefits, so we absolutely recommend ultrasound use in even the highest risk pregnancies, as long as it is performed by trained personnel in accredited facilities.

Ultrasound bonding

An emotional bond created between parents and the fetus when the fetus is viewed by ultrasound.

SECOND TRIMESTER

In the second trimester, the baby's organ systems have become fully developed, and from here forward, the fetus grows primarily in size and weight. By now, the fetus's heartbeat should be distinctly audible on a handheld Doppler. Fetal movement is usually felt for the first time between 18 and 22 weeks, particularly in women who've had children before. If you don't feel anything, that's not necessarily an indication that something is wrong—it likely means that your baby's movements are cushioned by the placenta (particularly if the placenta is attached at the anterior, or back, end of the uterus). Meanwhile, for the mother, this period usually represents a transition to an easier, more enjoyable part of the pregnancy. The mother usually has more energy, and many of the symptoms of the first trimester decrease or disappear altogether as levels of hCG decline.

Between 15 and 20 weeks of gestation, the **maternal serum alpha-fetoprotein (MSAFP)** test is administered as part of **second trimester screening**. This test measures levels of alpha-fetoprotein (AFP), a substance produced by the liver of the fetus, in the mother's bloodstream to determine whether there is a risk of "open" birth defects—abnormalities in which specific structures in the fetus don't close properly, causing the fetus to leak AFP, such as neural tube defects, abdominal wall defects, or kidney disorders. The MSAFP test is commonly performed in conjunction with measurements of levels of hCG, estriol, and inhibin, as the levels of these hormones can indicate potential problems that can be explored through further prenatal testing (see Question 9). The screening process for these hormones is commonly called a **quad screen**.

Second trimester screening also calls for an **ultrasound fetal survey** at about 18 weeks. A specialist trained in fetal ultrasonography will look at the fetus's organs, record its heart rate, measure its bones, and review its overall position within the uterus, checking the position and blood-flow status of

The Basics

Maternal serum alpha-fetoprotein (MSAFP)
A blood test measuring levels of alpha-fetoprotein to assess the risk of certain birth defects.

Second trimester screening
A series of tests, including ultrasound and the "quad screen" used to determine the risk of birth defects, especially neural tube defects.

Quad screen
Screening for levels of four key hormones—MSAFP, hCG, estriol, and inhibin—that if abnormal can suggest potential problems with a pregnancy.

Ultrasound fetal survey
An ultrasound examination of the physical status and position of the fetus, umbilical cord, and placenta.

the placenta. If the parents request it—and if the baby co-operates—the specialist can also try to determine the baby's gender. The fetal survey is probably the first place that any abnormalities in the pregnancy will show up, including multiple fetuses; therefore, the ultrasound is often the starting point in addressing any problems. However, the ability to detect birth defects by ultrasound is not 100% accurate but varies depending on how experienced the specialists are and how up-to-date their equipment is.

Elizabeth's comment:

The first fetal survey is a mixed bag when you are a "high-risk" mother. On one hand, it's incredibly exciting when all of the fatigue and the nausea suddenly coalesce into an actual, visible, tangible being. At the same time, you're holding your breath because you know that you're high risk. Initially, I was concerned that they'd find twins, as my age, weight, family history of twins, and use of fertility drugs all greatly increased my chances of multiples. Twins may be double the joy, but they're also double the workload. At the time, I was supporting my family while my husband built our house—twins would have meant that I might have to leave my job. When I saw my solo fetus on the monitor, one worry was taken off my mind. My son was normal in all respects, and I felt a great deal more positive. Nevertheless, I was still concerned, as the ultrasound showed partial placenta previa. My doctor reassured me that the problem would likely resolve itself; thus, I tried to focus on the fact that I had a healthy baby instead of being anxious about possibly needing a cesarean. Worry is the hardest part about carrying the "high-risk" label.

THIRD TRIMESTER

During the final 3 months of the pregnancy, many changes occur as a result of both the baby's rapid growth and the body's preparations for birth. The cocktail of hormones that was released in earlier stages changes somewhat in composition as hormones that regulate birth and milk production are released in greater amounts, while production of certain other hormones decreases. The placenta releases **corticotrophin-releasing hormone** to signal that the pregnancy is nearing its end and to stimulate various changes in the pituitary glands and the uterus that need to occur before birth can take place. A decline in progesterone levels, meanwhile, means that this hormone's role in preventing uterine contractions is diminished, and the mother begins to experience **Braxton-Hicks contractions** as "practice" for labor (see Question 59). Another hormone, **relaxin**, softens and enlarges the cervix and relaxes ligaments to assist the passage of the infant through the birth canal.

At the same time, the kicking, squirming, punching, hiccuping, and other sensations that the mother experiences slow because the baby has started to run out of room to maneuver. Because the baby can still move about, the mother should still feel regular sensations telling her that the baby is awake and active. Near the very end of the pregnancy, the baby "drops"—that is, assumes a head-down position within the cradle of the pelvis. Finally, the mother begins to experience the symptoms of labor—regular, repeated, painful, and steady contractions and the less obvious symptoms of effacement (shortening) and dilation (opening) of the cervix (as determined by a doctor's examination).

Pregnancies that were completely normal throughout may end in a difficult and complicated labor or a **cesarean section**; complicated pregnancies sometimes finish on a high note with a "textbook" delivery of a healthy baby. Although some situations can predetermine a nonstandard birth process (for example, conditions such as placenta previa; see Question 83), most of the time, the duration of labor and difficulty of delivery are impossible to predict. Those few "predictable" labor and delivery complications are addressed in Questions 55 and 83.

Corticotrophin-releasing hormone

A hormone released by the placenta near the end of the pregnancy to stimulate changes that precede delivery.

Braxton-Hicks contractions

Contractions occurring before labor that function as "practice" for the uterus.

Relaxin

A hormone that causes loosening of ligaments and cervical ripening prior to labor.

Cesarean section

Surgery to extract the fetus from the uterus through the abdomen when vaginal birth is not possible or dangerous.

The Basics

2. What problems can occur in pregnancy?

Situations that can turn a normal pregnancy into a complicated one can be divided into three types:

1. Complications caused by an abnormal response of the mother's body to pregnancy-induced changes—including situations in which a preexisting health problem interferes with the mother's physiological condition as the pregnancy progresses. Diabetes, cardiovascular disease, thyroid dysfunction, pulmonary disease, and similar conditions can have a strong impact on the baby's health and development. Alcohol use, smoking, drug abuse, eating disorders, and similar "external" factors are bad for the baby's proper development; these should be regarded as preexisting maternal health problems, even when the mother's health doesn't seem to be directly affected by them. Underlying problems in the mother don't always directly harm the baby, but if the mother's health worsens during pregnancy, it is generally bad for the baby as well.

2. Complications stemming from atypical development in the baby. Such complications generally affect the physical welfare of the mother much less, but they can cause significant health problems in the baby and may even lead to miscarriage, premature delivery, or stillbirth. "Atypical development" is a catchphrase that includes not only serious abnormalities, such as genetic and congenital disorders, but also more benign situations, such as twin or multiple fetuses, which technically aren't "abnormal" unless some other factor is at play (conjoined twins, for example, but see Questions 36 and 37 for more on the subject of multiples). However, multiple pregnancies nonetheless are not considered "typical" of a normal pregnancy, and the risk of complications is higher with more than one fetus.

3. Complications related to labor and delivery, including preterm labor, placenta previa, and other situations that

can affect otherwise normal pregnancies. In these situations, a healthy mother and baby are at risk for complications at the beginning of or during labor and delivery.

The presence of any one of these complications does not preclude another from occurring, and in some situations, the presence of one type of complication might make others even more likely. Mothers carrying twins or multiples, for example, have a higher likelihood of preterm labor and other delivery-related complications than mothers of single babies.

Whether you're at risk for any of these types of complications depends on a combination of many factors. Your age, your personal health history, and your familial health history are the three most important factors, as they directly affect potential risk levels. To a smaller extent, your ethnic background can sometimes increase your risk of specific conditions, even if you have no family history of them. Also, the place where you live, your level of education, and your financial situation can sometimes affect your access to health care before and during your pregnancy, which in turn has an impact on the risk level for certain complications and, more importantly, the final outcome of the complications. If you live in a rural area where the nearest hospital is over an hour away and does not have a neonatal intensive care facility, for example, your risk of preterm labor may not change, but the chance of having a poor outcome increases if your baby is very premature.

Your doctor and nurse(s) are most likely to have accurate information at their fingertips, so trust them—but be sure you don't let your anxieties get in the way of hearing what they say. If they tell you that there's a greater risk of a specific problem arising because of your personal health history, you may feel anxious or worried, but remember that "greater" is a relative term. For example, for an average 25-year-old woman, the risk of having a child with Down syndrome is about 1 in 1,250; for an average 40-year-old woman, the risk is about 1 in 106. The 40-year-old woman has a risk factor that is more than 10 times greater than the 25-year-old woman, with all other aspects being equal. This sounds scary if you look at just that statistic alone—nevertheless, the 40-year-old woman's chance of actually *having* a baby with Down syndrome is still less than 1%. Most people would consider that a pretty low risk! Thus, be sure that you get clear information from your health care providers about exactly what your "increased" risk means for you overall and, more important, whether there's anything that you can do to minimize this risk.

3. Why is my pregnancy considered high risk?

A pregnancy can be classified as *high risk* for a number of reasons. The most common reason is the age of the mother: A woman who is older than age 35 (see Question 17) or younger than age 18 has a greater chance of experiencing complications in the pregnancy or at birth. Preterm labor and low-birthweight babies are particular problems for adolescent mothers, whose bodies often are not yet fully mature and therefore are less well equipped to handle the burden of pregnancy. Older mothers, on the other hand, are at greater risk for a host of complications: for example, high blood pressure, miscarriage, gestational diabetes, chromosomal abnormalities in the baby, and multiple pregnancies. Particularly for older mothers having their first child, complications such as **placenta previa** or **placental abruption** (see Questions 42 and 43) are more likely to occur than in younger mothers or mothers with prior pregnancies.

A preexisting health problem in the mother, no matter the age, is the next most common reason for categorizing a pregnancy as high risk. Although even seemingly minor issues can have adverse effects on the pregnancy or the baby's health—smoking or drinking alcohol, for example, can cause a number of health problems to the fetus, even if done on a casual or occasional basis (see Question 20)—a significant medical problem in the mother is usually sufficient to categorize her pregnancy as high risk. Such problems include **chronic** endocrine disorders such

---

Placenta previa

A condition in which the placenta partially or completely covers the cervix.

Placental abruption

A condition in which the placenta has pulled away from the wall of the uterus prior to birth.

Chronic

Long-term, ongoing disorders or conditions.

as diabetes (see Question 25), autoimmune disorders such as multiple sclerosis or lupus erythematosus (see Question 26), cancer, whether active or in remission (Question 28), certain infectious diseases, including sexually transmitted diseases (Question 29), and the use of (or need for) infertility treatment to get pregnant (Question 31). All of these situations are common in both younger and older women, and all would cause a pregnancy to be considered high risk. It is less common for the high risk to stem from a problem with the baby. If either parent has a family history of certain **congenital** disorders or known **genetic mutations**, the pregnancy is generally assumed to have a higher risk of potential complications related to the baby's welfare. Certain screening tests, as described in Question 1, may suggest potential risk factors when there are no known congenital or genetic risks. A positive result in a screening test may justify a change in status to "high risk," or it may simply trigger a second round of testing before that designation is applied. Either way, it helps to be fully informed about what the screening test looks for and its accuracy before assuming that your heightened risk level is cause for concern.

Congenital
Present before birth.

Genetic mutations
Alterations to DNA that occur randomly.

Finally, a pregnancy might be labeled high risk because of unusual circumstances affecting the support system for the fetus—the uterus, placenta, umbilical cord, and amniotic sac. A number of conditions that might affect the welfare of the fetus are related to how blood flows from mother to fetus through the placenta and umbilical cord, as well as situations related to the amniotic sac and surrounding fluids. Some of these tend to occur most often in older and/or first-time mothers but can happen to just about anyone, even mothers who have had uncomplicated previous pregnancies. Such situations are described further in Questions 40–44.

Elizabeth's comment:

Because I got pregnant for the first time at the age of 37, I knew that I was high risk. I thought that the risk was primarily because

*of the increased likelihood of having a child with Down syndrome.
I knew almost nothing about the many other potential complications, whether associated with "advanced maternal age" or not.
My first ultrasound, however, showed a complication—partial
placenta previa. This put me squarely in the high-risk category,
even without considering my age. My doctor assured me that this
could resolve itself over the course of the pregnancy, and it did . . .
just in time for pregnancy-induced hypertension, another common
complication in older first-time mothers. My age and about 35
pounds of excess weight aside, I was in relatively good health before
getting pregnant, so I never thought about my own welfare—all of
my worries up to that point had been focused on having a healthy
baby boy. As it turned out, he was strong, active, and completely
normal; instead, I was the one with the health problems! This situation was opposite from everything that I'd ever assumed about
high-risk pregnancies.*

4. Who is most at risk in a high-risk pregnancy: me or my baby?

The easy answer to this question is that the baby is most at
risk, as some complications can harm the baby without affecting the mother, but nearly all complications that affect
the mother's health have the possibility of either directly or
indirectly harming the baby.

Most of the time, the complications in a high-risk pregnancy
are related to the mother's health. In these cases, the goal
becomes keeping the mother's physical welfare stable long
enough for her to give birth to a baby who is capable of living outside of the womb. The key to success is to find ways to
manage the mother's health so that she isn't greatly harmed
for the longest possible duration of the pregnancy; the birth
of the baby often clears up the complication, unless it was a
previously existing or hidden health problem. Ideally, the
baby's stay in the uterus should be prolonged so that the
mother can give birth normally; however, this isn't always
possible—for instance, if the mother's health becomes

critical before the baby is full term, the medical team must assess whether the baby has developed enough to survive with assistance. If so, then labor may be **induced** early so that the baby is born prematurely and cared for in a **neonatal intensive care unit (NICU)** (see Question 84 for more about inducing premature birth). In some circumstances, a cesarean section might be required—for example, if the baby is not strong enough to withstand the stress of vaginal birth or if a vaginal birth should be avoided (see Question 83). If the baby is developed enough to survive, the health care team must then help the parents understand that they are likely to lose the pregnancy or—under extreme and very rare circumstances, such as ectopic pregnancy, or severe maternal illness, such as pulmonary hypertension—that they must terminate the pregnancy in order to preserve the mother's health or life (see Question 85).

The management of a pregnancy complicated by maternal health problems is generally determined on a case-by-case basis. **Bed rest** is commonly used to treat a variety of complications (see Question 80), as it reduces some of the physical stresses on the body. Bed rest, however, is often prescribed when it isn't really necessary, and some complications can arise with strict bed rest that could make matters worse (Question 81). Management of diet and nutrition and fetal monitoring are key factors in handling most maternal health problems. Medications are used in some situations, but in others, they tend to be the final solution because they have not been adequately tested in pregnant women. Often there's no way of knowing exactly what effects they might have on a developing fetus, particularly in the early stages of pregnancy. Medications for preexisting health conditions such as thyroid disorders, diabetes, or epilepsy may need to be reevaluated during pregnancy because the changes in the mother's body may require a different dose.

The Basics

Induced

Caused to occur artificially.

Neonatal intensive care unit (NICU)

A specialized facility in a hospital where ill or premature babies are cared for.

Bed rest

A prescription requiring a patient to rest in bed part or all of the day as well as night.

Management of diet and nutrition and fetal monitoring are key factors in handling most maternal health problems.

When the mother is healthy but the baby is not, the method of handling the situation is often similar in its goal—keeping the baby in utero as long as possible—which sometimes requires rather complicated strategies. Many congenital birth defects can be detected via ultrasound and a few can be corrected surgically even while the baby is still in the uterus (see Question 35). In most situations, surgery is performed hours, days, or weeks after the baby is born, and in some, corrective measures may require years, although immediate steps are taken to ensure that the infant has adequate oxygen and nutrition via gastrostomy (stomach) or endotracheal (airway) tubes. It is most important, however, to simply have the equipment and staff needed to care for the baby immediately after birth.

There's no way to look at any woman and say that she definitely will or won't have complications.

5. Is there any way to predict who will or won't have complications?

Predispose

Having an increased risk.

In some cases, certain factors **predispose** a woman to having complications (see Question 3), but for the most part, there's no way to look at any woman and say that she definitely will or won't. It is best to collect as much information as possible about the mother's health, including her history and her family and partner's histories, perform the appropriate screening and **prenatal testing** (see Questions 9–16), and use all of this collected information to make an estimation of whether particular problems may arise. The steps that can be taken to reduce the risk of complications are discussed in Question 8.

Prenatal testing

A collection of diagnostic tests that can suggest or confirm disorders in the fetus.

Population studies

Research that examines large groups of people to determine what proportion of the population may experience certain phenomena.

6. How does my physician determine my risk for complications?

As we stated in Question 1, *risk* is the likelihood of a particular event happening under particular circumstances. This is calculated by determining how often such an event occurs in similar people in similar circumstances. In medicine, this determination is made through **population studies**, which track a collection of individuals with specific similarities (such as gender, age, and race) for a set period of time to determine how many experience a particular health event. For example, if a group of 1,000 women who are 40 years old are watched for 5 years and if 21 of them fall ill with a particular lung disease, one could conclude that the risk of this lung disease in a woman age 40 to 45 is approximately 21 in 1,000 (2.1%). This **statistic** is a snapshot of risk; the more individuals are included in the population, the more accurate the statistic will be.

Your doctor will ask you to describe your personal and familial health history in detail. This will determine your personal likelihood of experiencing various complications. He or she will also perform the baseline tests described in Question 1. Using the information from your history and the tests, your doctor will make an assessment about where you fit in with the statistics for specific problems. If your doctor finds a heightened risk for complications, he or she will investigate further or, if appropriate, will try to prevent or alleviate the condition(s) that causes concern.

You can generally trust your doctor and nurses to give you accurate information. However, some women prefer to research their own health situation themselves, and we encourage that. An informed patient can take better care of herself. There is one warning we would offer, however: If you look up your condition on the web or in the library, you will find that there is a lot of information available. Some of it is good information based on studies including a lot of women, but other information isn't as good. It can be hard to tell which sources are correct, especially when the information is confusing or frightening. Here are some rules of thumb to help you weed out the good from the bad. First, look to see where the original information comes from. If you read an article that refers to studies in medical journals, such as the *American Journal of Obstetrics and Gynecology*, the information probably is accurate. If the article relates a "first-hand experience" or talks

Statistic

A numerical summation of data collected during research.

to only one "expert" without giving alternative points of view, however, treat it with skepticism—such stories are written more to attract attention than to pass on real information. Reports in the mass media often contain inaccuracies, so don't be surprised if your doctor downplays the importance of an article that you read in *USA Today*—it's likely that the article didn't give the full picture, and your doctor knows it. Second, turn to governmental agencies such as the National Institutes of Health and academic institutions and teaching hospitals. Many of these sources have patient outreach and education programs you can contact for more information.

Take what you read with a grain of salt, and discuss your concerns with your doctor.

Be wary of information that isn't backed up by widely accepted research, as such information abounds on the Internet and in mass media. Take what you read with a grain of salt, and discuss your concerns with your doctor. Remember that your doctor likely sees these situations on a daily basis, and he or she knows best whether they apply to your situation.

7. Will my OB/GYN know how to treat my condition, or do I need to see a specialist?

Most OB/GYNs are qualified to handle high-risk pregnancies. Many factors that turn an ordinary pregnancy into a high-risk situation are relatively common, so an experienced OB/GYN has seen them before and will know how to treat them. More importantly, your OB/GYN is familiar with *you* and therefore should have a better understanding of your overall health than someone with whom you have no long-term relationship. Doctors are not magicians or mind readers, and familiarity with a patient's history counts for a lot during treatment. It's therefore not necessary, or even a good idea, to switch to a specialist simply because your pregnancy is high risk.

Maternal/fetal medicine specialist

A physician specializing in treatment of high-risk pregnancies.

In some circumstances, however, a **maternal/fetal medicine specialist** (formerly called a **perinatologist**)—or even a team of specialists—is necessary. If multiple risk factors affect your pregnancy or if the complications are particularly serious or unusual, the assistance of a doctor whose principal focus is high-risk pregnancy might tip the balance in your favor. For the most part, your own OB/GYN will probably refer you to such a specialist if necessary, but if you are concerned that the care you're receiving may not be enough given the risks, don't hesitate to ask your doctor for a referral to a specialist. One warning on that front: specialists in high-risk obstetrics are not always available. For example, if you don't live near a big city with a major medical center, you may not have easy access to a specialist who handles high-risk pregnancy. Various organizations listed in the Appendix (under the *Specialist Listings* heading) can help you find the nearest specialist; however, you may need to travel a long distance, and this stress might do as much harm as the specialist could do you good. If this is the case and your condition is serious enough to require a specialist, talk to your OB/GYN about long-distance consultation—your doctor may be able to coordinate your care with the specialist, limiting your need for travel.

If complications are particularly serious or unusual, a doctor whose principal focus is high-risk pregnancy might tip the balance in your favor.

8. If I am already pregnant, is there any way that I can reduce the risk or alter any of the risk factors?

You can't do anything about some risk factors—age and genetics, for instance—but you can reduce the risk of many complications (and some birth defects) by improving your overall health. When stronger and healthier, you generally have a greater chance of preventing and/or successfully overcoming potential complications. Also, a healthier mother tends to give birth to a healthier baby. Obviously, health improvements are best made before pregnancy, but even while pregnant it's not too late to make changes that will reduce the risk for a number of complications.

Even if you're already pregnant, it's not too late to make changes that will reduce the risk for complications.

Some of the things you can do are commonsense changes. If you smoke, quit. Ask your doctor to help—you *can* do it, and the sooner you start, the better (though we know that it will not be fun). Likewise, eliminate the use of alcohol and recreational drugs altogether. If this is difficult because you have an **addiction,** be honest with your doctor; he or she will help you to address the problem. Read Question 20 so that you'll understand the serious side effects of drug and alcohol use.

Also, get at least 8 hours of sleep every night, as this is crucial for maintaining good health. Most people don't get enough, even without the added stress of pregnancy. If the usual discomforts of pregnancy interfere with nighttime sleep, take a nap in the afternoon to restore some of your energy. Resist the temptation to stay up watching television or reading a book, as this sleep loss can make you cranky and tired and can alter your metabolism. No studies are available to detail the specific effects of sleep loss on pregnant women, but studies of habitual sleep loss in general show that sleeping too little seems to promote higher glucose levels in the bloodstream. People seem to become more glucose resistant, and therefore more prone to diabetes, if they sleep less. Given that pregnancy itself can sometimes cause a temporary form of diabetes (see Questions 50–52), a pregnant woman does not want to do anything that increases that possibility.

Also, most people don't get enough fluids, meaning water or juice (but mostly water). Cut back on caffeinated beverages such as coffee or cola (eliminate them entirely, if possible), and start drinking water instead. Yes, it means more trips to the bathroom, but drinking water benefits you and your baby in many ways, including maintaining energy. Pregnancy hormones affect the way your body uses and stores fluids; you probably have already realized that you urinate more while pregnant. This increase means that pregnant women are more susceptible to **dehydration.** By drinking between 48 and 64 ounces of water daily, or approximately three of the standard bottles you can buy at a vending machine, you can prevent both minor problems, such as dry skin and constipation, and possibly some major ones, including preterm labor, which is

Addiction

Inability to control or stop the use of alcohol, tobacco, illegal drugs, or prescription medications.

Drinking between 48 and 64 ounces of water daily can prevent both minor problems and possibly some major ones, including preterm labor.

Dehydration

Insufficient water intake, leading to too little fluid in the body.

sometimes brought on by dehydration. Caffeine, a natural diuretic that promotes water loss (as well as potentially robbing you of badly needed sleep), should be avoided as much as possible.

Along with fluids, good nutrition is essential. Pregnant women need more of everything—that old cliché about "eating for two" is quite true—but in particular, they need more of the vitamins and minerals (especially calcium, iron, folic acid, and vitamin D), which are the "building blocks" for healthy bones and organs in their baby. Suggestions about healthy eating are found in Question 18, and Questions 67 and 68 discuss the importance of specific vitamins and minerals in pregnancy.

If you're not pregnant, exercise is important in helping you to prepare for pregnancy (and, if you're overweight, losing weight will help to prevent complications). Even if you *are* already pregnant, exercise prevents problems. Yes, women who are pregnant are told to "take it easy," and certainly, you do not need to take up kickboxing or aerobics if it's not something that you're already doing regularly; however, taking a 10- or 20-minute walk every few hours would help your circulation, improve your overall energy level, and generally do you good. If you have access to a swimming pool, use it; swimming is one of the best ways to get exercise during pregnancy because the water supports your weight and alleviates stress on your joints. Gentle forms of exercise that emphasize stretching and meditation, such as yoga and tai chi, are also beneficial (see Question 93). You should avoid certain exercises during pregnancy (see Question 70). Do not begin a new fitness routine (or add to an existing one) while you're pregnant, but if you are already accustomed to regular exercise, in most cases it's okay to continue, with a doctor's permission, at the same or slightly reduced levels of exertion. If you're not accustomed to regular exercise, introducing low-level, regular exercise such as swimming, yoga, or walking could help your energy levels—unless you have a complication, such as incompetent cervix (see Question 23), that would preclude exercise.

The Basics

Get enough rest, take time to relax, and be good to yourself.

Finally, take it easy! Get enough rest, take time to relax, and be good to yourself. Stress is inherent in a high-risk pregnancy, but any stress reduction is helpful . . . as long as it's a healthy technique. We're not advocating binge eating, chain smoking, or using drugs or alcohol to help you relax! Instead, you might want to go for a walk in a park, read a book, see a movie, get takeout, get a haircut, have your nails done, and get a massage. Little, special treats like this can sometimes lower your stress level and lessen your risk of complications.

PART TWO

Prenatal Testing

What is prenatal testing? When are more specialized
prenatal tests needed?

What are the benefits of prenatal testing?
Will testing help reduce my risk of problems
in pregnancy?

What prenatal tests are available? What do
they show?

More . . .

Down syndrome

A chromosomal abnormality (trisomy 21) that leads to variable levels of mental retardation and physical defects.

Edwards syndrome

A chromosomal abnormality (trisomy 18) causing severe physical defects that are often fatal.

Neural tube defects

Birth defects affecting the development of the spine and/or brain.

Amniocentesis

Collection of fetal cells using a needle guided into the amniotic sac.

Preterm labor

Labor that begins prior to the 37th week of pregnancy.

Intrauterine growth restriction (IUGR)

A condition in which a fetus does not grow at the rate normally expected.

Stillbirth

Death of the fetus after the 20th week of pregnancy.

9. What is prenatal testing? When are more specialized prenatal tests needed?

Prenatal testing is any type of blood work or imaging that can predict or diagnose either potential pregnancy complications or possible abnormalities in an unborn fetus. Although it includes the standard tests listed in Question 1, a collection of targeted tests are used to determine the likelihood of specific genetic or congenital abnormalities in the fetus. Such non-routine prenatal genetic tests may look for specific mutations that are associated with health problems, such as cystic fibrosis or major chromosomal errors such as Down syndrome. Other specialized prenatal tests target potential congenital birth defects such as cleft palate, certain heart defects, neural tube defects, and similar problems in the fetus.

Specialized prenatal testing is generally called for when one of the standard test results indicates a possible abnormality or when the mother or father's medical history points to an increased likelihood of a genetic syndrome (see Table 5 in Question 38). For example, when the MSAFP test returns a low AFP level in combination with abnormal levels of hCG, estriol, or inhibin, these results sometimes suggest that the baby has an increased risk of a chromosomal abnormality such as **Down syndrome** (also called trisomy 21) or **Edwards syndrome** (trisomy 18). Abnormal MSAFP results can also point to **neural tube defects** such as spina bifida. In either case, abnormal results might mean that further testing by a more advanced ultrasound and/or invasive methods such as **amniocentesis** would be appropriate, as these can often pinpoint for certain whether such abnormalities are indeed present.

Abnormal results in the MSAFP test can also indicate a risk for **preterm labor** (Questions 53 and 54), **intrauterine growth restriction (IUGR)** (Question 40), or **stillbirth** (Question 97), which alerts the physician to monitor the fetus more closely. Results from blood or imaging tests considered in combination with the MSAFP results could lead to more aggressive treatment plans when warranted. Usually such decisions are made on a case-by-case basis and depend on the health circumstances of both the fetus and the mother.

Even when the standard test results are completely normal, there are sometimes other reasons to test further. A mother may be referred for further testing if she or the father's family has one or more children born with a genetic birth defect, particularly if the problem is severe or life threatening to the fetus (see Question 38).

10. What are the benefits of prenatal testing? Will testing help reduce my risk of problems in pregnancy?

Prenatal testing provides two distinct benefits: First, it often rules out problems, which can relieve the parents' minds of anxiety, and second, discovering birth defects *before* the baby is born can allow for proper preparation. Prenatal testing probably will not reduce your overall risk, but it may give your doctor enough information to help reduce the severity of a problem. Some congenital heart and spine defects can be surgically repaired in utero (see Question 35), allowing the fetus to heal and continue developing in the enclosed security of the uterus. Even in situations in which there are no possible treatments before birth, knowing that a defect exists can allow the medical team to address the newborn's needs immediately after birth (see Question 15).

Many birth defects can be detected before birth but cannot be treated or changed. In these cases, prenatal testing lets the parents know what to expect when their baby is born. Having a baby with severe birth defects is extremely stressful, and although prenatal testing may not necessarily eliminate the problem, it can at least reduce the shock at the time of birth.

Elizabeth's comment:

My first OB/GYN suggested prenatal screening based solely on my age-related risk of chromosomal abnormalities. I'd looked up the statistics on Down syndrome and compared it with the statistics on complications related to amniocentesis; they were almost identical—meaning that the likelihood of having a positive test result was about the same as the chance of a serious problem occurring from the test itself. In fact, the chance of a test-related problem was slightly greater. I'd been trying to get pregnant for almost 2 years, and I wasn't willing to risk a complication simply to learn about a problem that I couldn't change. My doctor understood my reasoning and emotional reaction and didn't press the matter, although she did point out that knowing ahead of time about a child's special needs would give me more time to get used to the idea and to find services to help care for and educate the child; however, like any prospective mother, I really didn't even want to think about the possibility. Thankfully, my son turned out to be healthy. Nevertheless, she was right—if there had *been a problem, I'd have been completely unprepared for it at the time of his birth. Given that I had just come through 33 hours of very difficult, complicated labor, the impact on me in my exhausted state is unimaginable. For that reason, I made a different decision with my second child: I had the tests.*

11. What prenatal tests are available? What do they show?

Chorionic villus sampling

Collection of fetal cells from the placenta for diagnosis of chromosomal disorders.

Fundal height

Measurement of uterine expansion over the course of pregnancy.

Prenatal tests come in two forms: indirect testing, in which the fetus's welfare is determined by measuring whether the mother's body is changing along expected parameters, and direct testing of the fetus through ultrasound and other electronic monitors as well as by invasive techniques such as **chorionic villus sampling** and amniocentesis. Indirect techniques include measurement of **fundal height** (that is, the distance that the bulging uterus expands over time), monitoring of the mother's weight gain, and blood analysis to look for markers related to fetal abnormalities, as mentioned in Question 1. Direct techniques include ultrasound (particularly nuchal translucency scans, described in Question 14, and biophysical profiles), nonstress testing and heart rate monitoring, sampling of amniotic fluid, chorionic villus sampling, placental biopsy, and direct fetal blood sampling.

12. Are there any risks from the tests?

For most forms of prenatal testing, there is no risk to mother or fetus because the tests are noninvasive. Most of the tests described in earlier questions involve the use of ultrasound and/or blood screening, none of which directly impact the fetus or its surroundings. The only tests that hold any risk for the fetus are amniocentesis and chorionic villus sampling, which involve collecting cells from within the uterine environment. In the first instance, a sample of amniotic fluid is drawn from within the sac surrounding the fetus; in the second, tissue samples are taken from the placenta. In both cases, the samples must be collected using a long, ultrasound-guided needle, and like any invasive procedure, there is a small risk of harm to the fetus or loss of the pregnancy. Most doctors and pregnancy advice books put the risk of amniocentesis-related miscarriage at about 0.5% 1 in 200—but that figure is based on studies done in the 1970s. Decades of improvements in technology and technique suggest a far lower risk, perhaps as low as 1 in 1,000. Chorionic villus sampling is still a relatively new procedure and carries higher risk—approximately 1 in 100 pregnancies—but with technological improvements, that rate will likely decline over time.

Keep in mind, however, that these are *average* rates and do not reflect the different capabilities of different hospitals and technicians. A hospital equipped with state-of-the-art ultrasound and highly trained, experienced technicians and physicians is likely to have a much lower rate of complications in these tests than one that has older equipment or less experienced staff. Thus, it makes sense to "comparison shop" for the facility that has the equipment and the experience to minimize the chance of complications.

13. How do I know whether the tests are accurate?

The accuracy of the test depends on several factors: First, what type of test is it—a blood screen, an imaging scan, or a chromosomal analysis? Second, who is performing the test? Is the technician or physician experienced in interpreting the test results? Third, what kind of result does the test produce? Is the result an absolute (in which a distinct feature can be observed, such as a cell count or heartbeat), or is it an estimation (in which a measurement falls within or outside an expected normal range)? All of these factors are important when determining the accuracy of the test results.

Tests that rely on blood samples generally fall in the category of estimations, and the results found in a single sample should not be considered absolutely accurate. The composition of your blood (that is, the blood cell count, hormones, sugars, and so on that can be measured in the blood) is not static but varies as your personal circumstances change. For example, if a sample is taken when you haven't eaten in a while, your **glucose** (blood sugar) level may be considerably lower than if the sample is drawn a half hour after a big breakfast. Physicians sometimes try to control such variables when targeting a specific measurement; for example, when checking blood glucose levels, your doctor may ask you to refrain from eating the morning of the test. Some factors, however, cannot be controlled. If you're just recovering from a bad cold when the sample is taken, you may display a higher than normal white blood cell count. A lab technician who analyzes a blood sample may note this and suggest that your physician perform further testing to verify that it's not a more serious infection.

Glucose

Blood sugar.

Moreover, findings based on blood tests usually are not definitive diagnoses of a problem; instead, they merely suggest the presence of a problem. Just as an elevated white blood cell count can suggest the presence of an infection, the levels of certain hormones might suggest problems in various organs (the liver, for example); however, this doesn't mean that a problem actually exists—sometimes, levels of hormones that might be borderline or below the "normal" values are actually correct for that particular person. Normal values in medicine are an approximation and quite often are higher or lower than the individual's actual readings, even when that person is not suffering any ill health. For this reason, results from blood tests are usually not the foundation of a diagnosis unless they are clearly far outside of the norm and there is a specific, observable reason for the abnormality.

Imaging scans can show many details that blood tests can't, and in the hands of an experienced specialist, imaging tests such as ultrasound can give a highly accurate profile that can be used for diagnoses. Scans, however, are only as "good" as the specialist performing them; an experienced, knowledge-able specialist is far more likely to have accurate results than one who is inexperienced. Many imaging units will have a novice technician shadow a more experienced staff member, thus eliminating the potential for error and raising the overall accuracy of imaging tests. Also, modern ultrasound, MRI, CT, and X-ray equipment continually improve, making these tests that much more accurate.

Karyotyping or chromosome analysis is by far the most accurate form of testing available . . . for *some* things. A karyotype that shows a chromosomal abnormality (such as trisomy 18 or trisomy 21) is considered to be nearly 100% accurate in diagnosing the associated syndrome (see Question 14). It will not tell you, however, whether the child will have physical and mental disabilities or how severe such disabilities might be. Some chromosomal abnormalities may not lead to any obvious physical or developmental characteristics—Klinefelter's syndrome, for example, often does not affect the outward appearance or behavior of the baby who has it and is invisible except in a chromosome analysis. Other abnormalities, such as Down syndrome, are characterized by physical or mental disabilities, but these can range from mild (where a child may

Karyotyping
Chromosome analysis.

Prenatal Testing

need some special educational assistance but is otherwise capable of functioning independently) to severe (where constant supervision and assistance are required because of severe mental and physical limitations). Chromosome analysis cannot currently predict where an individual baby will fall within this range. Furthermore, karyotyping does not detect mutations and errors at the level of individual genes. Many congenital disorders may occur because of as yet unknown genetic defects. Great strides have been made in this direction since a scientific program called the Human Genome Project succeeded in mapping all human genes in 2003; however, the specific functions of most genes are still known superficially at best, and the way that genes combine to cause (or prevent) human diseases, including genetic diseases, is poorly understood.

Ultimately, your physician and the staff nurse(s) are the best resources for understanding test results and their accuracy. Their job is to determine how the test results mesh with your specific circumstances. They also likely understand the capabilities of the technicians at the hospital or clinic where you are a patient. Thus, talk to your doctor or the nurses on staff about your concerns, and feel free to ask questions until you understand the information.

14. I've heard babies born to older mothers are at higher risk for Down syndrome. How do physicians test for Down syndrome? What do the test results mean?

Older mothers do face an increased risk of giving birth to a child with chromosomal abnormalities, including Down syndrome. For many years, the standard method of detecting such birth defects in utero has been amniocentesis. The amniotic fluid contains cells shed from the fetus (Figure 5); these cells can be isolated from the fluid. Chorionic villus sampling can also be used, although it is less commonly used, mainly because it's still relatively new. Chromosomes from these fetal cells are then examined for signs of abnormalities;

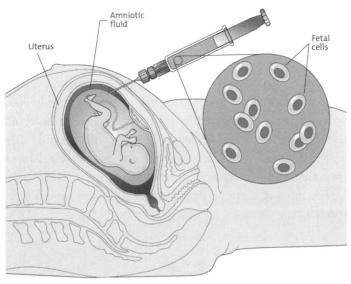

Figure 5   Amniocentesis.
SOURCE: Crowley, *An Introduction to Human Disease, Seventh Edition,* 2007: Jones and Bartlett Publishers LLC, Sudbury, MA. www.jbpub.com. Reprinted with permission.

Down syndrome, in particular, has a characteristic appearance of three copies of chromosome 21, instead of the usual pair.

Amniocentesis and chorionic villus sampling to examine fetal cells are the definitive diagnostic tools for Down syndrome and other chromosomal disorders, but they do have their drawbacks, primarily the risk of complications (see Question 12). Thus, other tests have been developed to estimate the probability of chromosomal disorders—then amniocentesis and chorionic villus sampling are used only when necessary. The most important of these is **first trimester screening**, in which an ultrasound is taken at 11 weeks to measure **fetal nuchal translucency**—that is, the size of a translucent space at the back of the baby's neck—in conjunction with blood drawn from the mother. The size of this translucent space, when looked at in combination with the blood test results, can give an accurate assessment of the risk of chromosomal abnormalities. If test results show an increased probability of chromosomal abnormalities, usually in the range of 1 in 220

First trimester screening

A screening test performed in weeks 11–14 that combines nuchal fold translucency with blood tests to look for chromosome abnormalities in the fetus.

Fetal nuchal translucency

The translucent space at the back of the fetus's neck.

or above, the obstetrician will likely suggest amniocentesis or chorionic villus sampling to see whether a chromosomal disorder is present. Where available, first-trimester screening to predict the presence of Down syndrome or other abnormalities is becoming a standard practice for both low- and high-risk mothers. The detection rate stands at roughly 90% accuracy when performed by experienced centers; however, relatively few technicians have been trained in this still fairly new technique, and it therefore isn't widely available. Moreover, the more experienced ultrasonographers tend to have higher rates of accurate detection than do less experienced specialists.

Elizabeth's comment:

In my first pregnancy, I refused testing for chromosomal anomalies; however, when my doctor discussed amniocentesis at the outset of my second pregnancy, I was more willing to listen. Because I still wasn't terribly excited about the idea of having a needle stuck into my belly, she suggested nuchal translucency screening. My doctor described this test to me as a noninvasive way of determining whether amniocentesis was really necessary. Although Cambridge Hospital didn't offer it, the hospital's Women's Health Center (of which my OB/GYN was chief) had formed a partnership with New England Medical Center, which did. Because of this partnership, my doctor could refer me for the test even though her own hospital didn't offer it. I was at 9 weeks, and therefore, we still had time to set up the appointments with the ultrasound technician and the genetic counselor. The tests were performed at 11 weeks, with a follow-up at 14 weeks. Hearing from the genetic counselor that the chance of my baby having a chromosomal abnormality was less than 1 in 1,000—when the average risk was about 1 in 90 for a woman my age—was worth all of the trouble of taking time off work and driving into downtown Boston.

15. If the prenatal tests show a problem with my health or with my baby, what can be done?

The possible approaches for handling prenatal complications depend on the complication. When the prenatal tests point to a problem with the health status of the mother, early intervention can resolve, or at least partially address, the problem. In many situations, treatments are available to either ensure a healthy baby and mom or at least minimize the effects on both. Specific strategies for differing complications are discussed in later questions, but in general, a pregnancy complicated by maternal health problems is handled as a balancing act—maintaining the mother's physical and emotional well-being while promoting development of the fetus for as long as possible in the womb. Neonatal intensive care facilities and prenatal surgery techniques may also be options when either the mother or the fetus has difficult problems that must be resolved before the baby reaches full term.

When the fetus has a health problem, the situation is more difficult. Some health problems have no solution: a chromosomal abnormality such as trisomy 18 (Edwards syndrome), for example, cannot be altered, and the grim outcome for the baby (severe birth defects leading to death by the age of 1 in almost all cases) cannot be changed at this time. In other cases, the baby's health problems can be resolved only through a difficult regimen of medical interventions—sometimes including surgeries and physical therapy—that may begin at or before birth and continue for months or even years. In still other cases, the health problem is such that no specific surgery or drug therapy can alter it, but a collection of educational and social interventions early in life can greatly improve the child's ability to function as he or she grows, so it is in the child's best interest to have such interventions available very soon after birth.

Although prenatal testing can identify these situations, the parents have the option of terminating the pregnancy—a heartbreaking decision under any circumstances (see Question 85)—or continuing the pregnancy. Many parents choose the second route. After this choice has been made, the strategy of the health care providers is threefold:

1. To support the mother's physical welfare to ensure that the baby is as physically robust as possible at birth
2. To assist the parents (and other family members) in coming to terms emotionally with the fact that the child will have ongoing and possibly significant health issues
3. To help the parents locate and establish a relationship with appropriate social service supports and to provide grief counseling and other services should the baby die (see Part Nine, Facing Loss in High-Risk Pregnancy)

Perhaps the greatest benefit of prenatal testing is that you are given advanced warning. Then you can prepare yourself for the emotional and financial stresses of either raising a child with mental or physical disabilities or having to say goodbye to that child soon after his or her birth. Many government and charitable agencies are available to assist the parents of special needs children; a listing of some agencies and organizations is available in the Appendix.

16. Is there any reason to refuse prenatal testing? How do I decide whether to get a test or refuse it?

Many women who are "high risk" refuse prenatal testing for various—often unspoken—reasons. Commonly, parents express concern that the tests could cause injury to the baby or that finding out about a birth defect might change the parents' feelings toward the unborn child. Some parents fear what they might learn, irrationally (but understandably) feeling that "ignorance is bliss" and "what we don't know won't hurt us." Others feel that the testing process causes anxiety, and they prefer to enjoy being pregnant without worrying about the rather remote possibility of a complication.

All of these reasons are valid emotional responses to a stressful situation, especially with a first child. We can counter each concern with facts and figures—stating, for example, that the chance of injury due to even the most invasive prenatal tests is less than 1 in 200 (0.5%) or that studies show that the vast majority of parents who have a child with a birth defect find that the child's disability does not interfere with the bond they develop with their child. The ultimate counterargument, however, is quite simply that ignorance is *not* bliss when it comes to the welfare of your baby. Sooner or later, the child will be born, and if he or she *does* have a health problem, the parents will need to make decisions immediately after the baby is born. Such decisions should be made when there is more time to think about the options. For example, for a child that will require assistance from social services, having sufficient lead time to coordinate health care, education, counseling, and other forms of assistance is very important. Bureaucracy does not move at the speed of parental need! Although the tests are worrisome, they will save you a great deal of stress if you find out about the problem before the baby's birth. Besides, if you find out that your baby is healthy, you will have relieved at least a part of the new-parent worry, high risk or not.

In the end, the decision to test or not test is the parents' choice. Doctors may advise you (possibly strongly) to get testing, but the final decision is up to you and your partner. Talk over all of the pros and cons with your partner and your doctor, and make sure that the decision that you come to is one that is best for you, your partner, and your baby.

PART THREE

Preexisting Risks: Mother's Health

Why am I considered to be "high risk" just because I'm over 35? How does my age affect my risk for complications?

I do a lot of running and sports, and my doctor told me I should cut back on some of my activities. Why? Isn't exercise good during pregnancy?

Why does my doctor think that I may be at risk for preterm labor or other complications?

More . . .

The wear and tear of age on the body affects its ability to respond to the demands of pregnancy.

17. Why am I considered to be "high risk" just because I'm over 35? How does my age affect my risk for complications?

Age does a number on our bodies: Our skin becomes less elastic, our bones more brittle, our muscles more susceptible to injury, and injuries take longer to heal. In general, our body systems work less effectively and less efficiently. For a pregnant woman who is over age 35, this means that the stress of pregnancy gets compounded because the body's systems don't bounce back as quickly. Thus, risk is increased primarily because the wear and tear of age on the body affects its ability to respond to the demands of pregnancy.

This wear and tear extends all the way down to the chromosomes. Women are born with their full complement of ova, which—just like the rest of our cells—deteriorate as we age. Older mothers have a higher risk of giving birth to babies with chromosomal abnormalities, of which Down syndrome is the best known, but not the only, birth defect; Figure 6 shows graphically just how sharply the risk level rises after age 35.

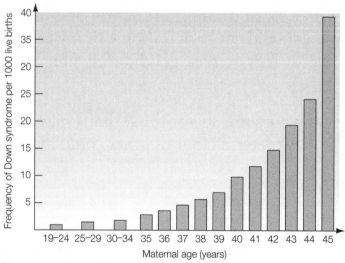

Figure 6   Incidence of Down syndrome babies at various maternal ages. The incidence of Down syndrome rises quickly after the maternal age of 35.
SOURCE: Chiras, *Human Biology, 5th Edition*, 2005: Jones and Bartlett Publishers LLC, Sudbury, MA. www.jbpub.com. Reprinted with permission.

There are a number of potential explanations for this situation, but the principal culprit is the abnormal division of older eggs, a phenomenon called **nondisjunction**. During nondisjunction, an egg undergoing division will receive an incorrect collection of chromosomes; the embryo that develops has either a greater or a lesser number of chromosomes than expected, leading to physical deformities, mental retardation, or even death. It's estimated that half of all fetuses with chromosomal abnormalities don't survive past the 12th week; the pregnancy ends in miscarriage. It is therefore no mere coincidence that older mothers have higher risk of both miscarriage *and* children born with birth defects. The simple truth is that the older the mother, the older the eggs, and the older the eggs, the greater the opportunity for abnormal development.

In addition, the hormonal changes and physical stresses of pregnancy sometimes bring out underlying conditions in the mother's physiology. Such conditions may range from the relatively benign—hypothyroid disease or mild diabetes, for example, which can have serious consequences for the baby but is fairly easy to treat (see Question 25)—to downright scary conditions such as breast cancer (the upsurge of estrogen in pregnancy can promote rapid development of certain estrogen-sensitive cancers). Older mothers also are more likely to have existing age-related diseases, including high blood pressure and cardiovascular disease, that when combined with the effects of pregnancy hormones can put them at risk for complications. Thus, the general statement that women older than 35 are "high risk" is based on the fact that time starts to have an impact on both reproduction capabilities and overall physical health.

Chronological age, however, is less important than **biophysical age**. A woman in her late 30s or 40s who is in good physical shape, is not overweight or underweight, eats a healthy diet low in fats and sugars, exercises regularly (but not to excess) (see Questions 19 and 70), does not smoke, drinks alcohol in

Nondisjunction

Abnormal division of a fertilized egg resulting in missing or extra chromosomes.

Biophysical age

Physical condition in comparison to the expected standard for the number of years one has lived.

Preexisting Risks: Mother's Health

47

moderation or not at all, and generally avoids stress will likely have just as good a chance at a complication-free pregnancy as a woman 5 or 10 years younger because these practices minimize wear and tear to the body. The estimations of who is at risk for certain age-related complications are based on an *average* women's health issues; if your physical health is better than average, your risk level is probably lower than average. Even though a woman over 35 has an increased risk of problems such as miscarriage, complications, and birth defects for the baby, the overall chances that any of these problems will arise are still fairly slim (as long as no other major health problems or known genetic syndromes are in her family history).

18. I was overweight before I became pregnant, and now there's no way to lose weight. Will this affect my risk for complications?

Yes, being overweight or obese does increase your risk of some complications. The most common pregnancy complications related to overweight and obesity are listed in Table 2.

Table 2   Common Pregnancy Complications Related to Overweight/Obesity

Maternal complications:
Gestational diabetes
Pregnancy-induced hypertension
Preeclampsia
Multiple fetuses
Fetal complications:
Difficulty monitoring fetal growth and development
Birth defects, particularly neural tube defects
Increased risk of miscarriage and stillbirth
Labor and delivery complications:
Increased risk of large-for-gestational age baby and longer, more difficult labor
Increased likelihood of cesarean coupled with greater risk of surgical complications
Longer post-delivery recovery time

A few of them may seem obvious—high blood pressure, for example—but you may be surprised to learn of certain other weight-related complications. An increased risk of twins and multiples, for example, has been found in overweight women. Many physicians counsel an overweight patient who is trying to become pregnant to lose weight before conceiving, and studies have even found that women who lose weight by gastric bypass surgery (a fairly extreme measure to combat severe obesity) end up with fewer complications in pregnancy than women who start their pregnancy severely overweight or obese. You'd think that having abdominal surgery would make you *more* prone to complications, but instead, this example simply reinforces the seriousness of excess weight for a pregnant woman.

What can be done if you're already pregnant? Most of the time, an overweight person can lose excess pounds by changing diet and exercise habits. More calories should be burned every day than the amount taken in. There is simply no other effective way to lose weight—but if you are already pregnant, that's exactly what you *can't* do. Your body needs adequate nutrition for both you *and* the baby, so caloric restriction is out of the question. If you're not already in an exercise program, starting one when you're under the physical strain of supporting a fetus is ill advised. In short, this is not the time to begin a new program of diet and exercise and *definitely* not the time to use any of the diet aids that are seen in magazines and on television! Also, you are obviously not a candidate for gastric bypass surgery at this point.

As a pregnant, overweight women, you have two goals: to minimize weight gain to no more than 10 to 15 pounds and to monitor your overall health. Your doctor may give you a referral to a nutritionist if your weight problem is especially severe to guide you in how to make choices that provide you and your baby with enough nutrients without adding extra calories. For the most part, however, you can take commonsense approaches to verify that you're eating enough without potentially adding to an existing weight problem.

- Stay well hydrated. Thirst and dehydration often masquerade as hunger; many people pack on excess pounds because they reach for snacks when their body really wants water. Keep water handy at all times, and if you feel hungry, drink 8 to 10 ounces. Then, if you're still hungry, eat something. *Do not* quench your thirst with sodas, juices, or sports drinks—they will simply add unnecessary calories. Avoid caffeinated drinks—they will make you more dehydrated, and studies have linked caffeine to an increased risk of miscarriage.
- Eat less food more often. First, this will help by preventing overpowering hunger so that you won't be inclined to overeat at mealtime. Second, as your baby grows, you will have less room for big meals anyway; therefore, habitually nibbling on small amounts of food will reduce the nausea, heartburn, or bloated feeling that can accompany a meal that is competing with your baby for belly space.
- Clear out junk food. This is a common and effective weight-loss strategy: If these high-calorie, low-nutrient foods aren't immediately available when you get hungry, you're less likely to eat them. Train yourself, and possibly your partner, to eliminate the usual suspects from the grocery cart. Make a grocery list before you head to the store, and then stick to it. If it's not on the list, don't put it in your cart. If it's not in your cart, it won't come home with you, and if it's not on your shelves at home, you're less likely to eat it at all, much less overindulge.
- Replace the bad with the better: look for a healthy snack food with similar qualities to a favorite unhealthy snack. Do you go for crunchy, salty chips? Substitute salted cucumber wedges or celery; the crunchy texture and salty taste may be what you're looking for. Do you like ice cream? Try low-fat frozen yogurt or fruit juice–based popsicles instead. Cookies? Look for the

brands that are specifically aimed for diabetics; they don't contain sugar and are generally lower in fats.

If you intend to have other children in the future, consult with your physician about weight loss before your next pregnancy. We also suggest breastfeeding your baby. The weight-loss benefits for the mother can be substantial and are worth considering.

Elizabeth's comment:

I started my first pregnancy 30 to 40 pounds overweight—heavy enough to qualify as "obese" by medical standards. I made a concerted effort to eat reasonably well and to take regular walks, and despite a very strong craving for chocolate milkshakes in the first and second trimesters (and bed rest during the third), I somehow managed to keep the weight gain to 20 pounds, a real accomplishment. During my second pregnancy, I started in better shape—I dropped 32 pounds after my son Nate was born, and I'd gotten myself into a better state of fitness. Although I was still about 25 pounds heavier than ideal, a greater portion of that weight was muscle instead of flab. I felt better; I had more energy and simply felt stronger. You can count me among the people who advocate breastfeeding, as it greatly helped my weight loss between pregnancies. I'm convinced that the weight loss is part of the reason I had fewer problems in my second pregnancy.

19. I do a lot of running and sports, and my doctor told me I should cut back on some of my activities. Why? Isn't exercise good during pregnancy?

In general, exercise *is* good during pregnancy, particularly if you are already physically fit. However, you probably will not be able to continue at your accustomed level of physical activity; 40% to 60% of a person's normal exercise levels are appropriate. Your heart rate should be kept to 140 beats per minute or less, and no more than 40 pounds should be lifted. Certain types of high-impact exercise are also not advisable because of stresses they put on your joints (see Question 70).

If you are underweight, your doctor may advise you to scale back on exercise. The type of high-end exercise regimen used by marathon runners or professional athletes, for example, tends to reduce body fat to levels below what is needed to support a pregnancy. This can be determined by looking at your height and weight on the Body Mass Index Table (available from the National Heart, Lung, and Blood Institute Web site, http://www.nhlbi.nih.gov/guidelines/obesity/bmi_tbl.htm). If your body mass index is below 18.5, you're underweight. Your doctor and nutritionist can advise you on appropriate ways to increase your weight—obviously, you could simply start eating massive amounts of high-fat foods, but the goal is to increase your weight *without* sacrificing nutrition! Furthermore, even if you are underweight, your doctor is not likely to want you to give up *all* exercise—after all, exercise during pregnancy is, in most cases, good for you and your baby.

Incompetent cervix

A cervix that is weak or thin and therefore opens prematurely during pregnancy.

For some conditions, even moderate exercise is a bad idea. Women with **incompetent cervix** (Question 23), for example, are often advised to give up all physical activity and may be put on bed rest for months at a time. You likely would already know this from having miscarried previously, which is usually how women discover that they have a weak cervix.

20. How does the use of illicit drugs, cigarettes, and alcohol affect pregnancy?

You probably have heard many of the cautions against using illicit drugs (including legal prescription medications used at improper doses or for reasons other than the prescribed use), alcohol, and cigarettes during pregnancy. How seriously you take them may depend on your attitude toward substance use in general; nevertheless, drug abuse, alcohol use, and tobacco use represent the leading *preventable* cause of birth defects and behavioral problems in infants and young children, according to the National Survey on Drug Use and Health (2005). Heavy use of *any* of these substances is likely to do harm to the fetus. The most common effects are low birthweight and poor **Apgar scores**; serious, sustained substance abuse may also lead to severe physical deformities, mental impairment, impaired vision, or lifelong behavioral problems—assuming, that is, that the pregnancy doesn't end in miscarriage or stillbirth, which is a much greater possibility in women with substance abuse problems. Occasional, moderate use of alcohol, tobacco, or illicit drugs may not harm your fetus; however, there is no guarantee that they won't, particularly if you already have other risk factors at play. Women experiencing a high-risk pregnancy should stay away from any use of alcohol, tobacco, or illicit drugs. The following information should explain why we make that recommendation.

Apgar scores

A series of tests after delivery that identify babies who have trouble adjusting to the outside environment.

ALCOHOL

In recent years, our society has grown increasingly aware of some of the negative aspects of substance use and abuse in pregnancy, but some of the information in general circulation, particularly about alcohol, can be confusing. On one hand, you may have been told that you should drink *no* alcohol at all; on the other, you may know mothers who drank alcohol in small amounts with no obvious ill effects on the baby. You may even know women who drank *a lot* while pregnant and still gave birth to a normal, healthy child. In the past, doctors have actually recommended a glass of wine to help pregnant women relax. So what is the true story?

Alcohol is a central nervous system depressant that has short-term toxic effects on brain cells and liver cells and long-term toxic effects on other body systems, such as the vascular system and the renal system (kidneys). Occasional alcohol use in a healthy, nonpregnant adult generally does not cause major health effects because the adult liver is able to process limited amounts of alcohol. The situation is different, however, for the fetus. Alcohol crosses the placental barrier easily, so it will quickly pass on to the fetus—but a fetus cannot process alcohol out of its liver and kidneys as fast as the mother can, so the glass of wine that gives her a mild buzz is the equivalent of a serious all-night bender for her baby.

The effects of alcohol on a fetus occur in a continuum called **fetal alcohol spectrum disorder**, ranging from minor behavioral and learning difficulties appearing during infancy and early childhood to a collection of serious mental and physical impairments known as **fetal alcohol syndrome**. Because alcohol is toxic to the central nervous system, the effects of alcohol are greatest in brain and nervous system development. Mental retardation, developmental and learning disabilities, poor motor coordination, hyperactivity, and sleep or sucking difficulties are common effects of heavy alcohol use during pregnancy. Growth during gestation and after birth is generally impaired, and in some cases, the baby will have a small head, low-set ears, a flat midface, and a short nose. The fetus may be so severely damaged that it dies before or at birth. Heavy alcohol use—that is, seven or more drinks per week and/or three or more drinks on multiple occasions during the pregnancy—has a 44% chance of causing fetal alcohol syndrome, with the remaining 56% falling somewhere farther in the spectrum of fetal alcohol effects.

Moderate or light use of alcohol during pregnancy is more difficult to quantify. In some cases, few noticeable effects are seen until many years later, when the child may show learning disorders or symptoms of ADHD—in other cases, there are no apparent effects at all. Because there is no way of knowing exactly how much will do harm, drinking any alcohol during pregnancy is risky. The recommendations from the U.S. Surgeon General, Centers for Disease Control, and many other sources of health data state that "no amount of alcohol can be considered safe" and that pregnant women should not drink alcohol at all. These organizations even say that women who might become pregnant—that is, women of childbearing age

---

Fetal alcohol spectrum disorder

A collection of physical effects on the fetus caused by alcohol consumption during pregnancy.

Fetal alcohol syndrome

Significant physical and mental impairment caused by high levels of alcohol consumption during pregnancy.

Drinking any alcohol during pregnancy is risky.

---

who are not using an effective form of birth control—should not drink alcohol at all if they are sexually active.

The Centers for Disease Control say that it's never too late to stop—the sooner, the better. This information may sound scary if you drank beer or wine about the time of conception. If you used alcohol before finding out you were pregnant, don't be overly alarmed—but stop using alcohol immediately now that you know you're pregnant.

TOBACCO

Like alcohol use, smoking during pregnancy directly affects the fetus in a number of ways. Toxins from tobacco smoke enter the placenta and interfere with the passage of oxygen and nutrients to the fetus; thus, the effects of tobacco use on the baby include poor prenatal growth, premature birth, an increased likelihood of stillbirth and infant death, as well as (less frequently) physical deformities such as cleft lip/palate, deformed fingers and toes, polycystic kidneys, defects of the aorta and pulmonary artery, defects of the abdominal wall, and skull deformation. Most of these abnormalities seem to be directly related to the effects of the **carbon monoxide** in cigarette smoke, but any of the 2,000 or so other chemicals present in cigarette smoke—many of them known toxins and cancer-causing agents—may also play a role. At least one study has suggested that nicotine alone (whether obtained in cigarette smoke or through other means, such as patches) can increase the risk of **sudden infant death syndrome (SIDS)** in newborns. Furthermore, smoking also greatly increases the risk of placenta previa and placental abruption (see Questions 42 and 43), and it may also increase the possibility of premature rupture of membranes.

Carbon monoxide

A toxin found in cigarette smoke and car exhaust.

Sudden infant death syndrome (SIDS)

Unexplained sudden death of a newborn or very young child.

There is some positive news on smoking and pregnancy. First, quitting smoking provides an *immediate* benefit to both the mother and the fetus. A woman who smokes through her first trimester but quits at the beginning of the second will probably have a baby of normal birthweight and few or no other health problems and will lower her risk of serious complications through the remainder of the pregnancy. As with alcohol, we encourage quitting at any point in the pregnancy (although earlier is better), not only because it will improve the overall health of mother and baby, but also because it increases the likelihood that the mother can maintain a smoke-free home after birth (thereby preventing a multitude of infant health problems, such as asthma, ear infections, and sleep disturbances). Second, you can use a nicotine patch to quit, but only if you do not continue to smoke while using the patch.

ILLICIT DRUGS

If we were to go into detail about the effects of every illegal drug available, this book would be many hundreds of pages, and we would leave out many legal drugs, such as painkillers, muscle relaxants, and antidepressants, that may be abused too. Street drugs such as marijuana, methamphetamine, ecstasy, cocaine/crack, heroin, and so on are linked to various birth defects, low birthweight, premature delivery, placental abruption, SIDS, and stillbirth. It is hard to state with any accuracy the extent to which a particular drug endangers the fetus because in many cases street drugs are used in combination with alcohol and/or tobacco. Moreover, given the nature of these illegal drugs, performing clinical or even animal trials to determine what sort of injury the drugs do to an unborn baby is out of the question; however, given the serious, even lethal, effects that these drugs often have on adult users, they likely would have similar and possibly greater effects on the fetus.

Legal drugs used in an illicit fashion may have a slightly better outcome in pregnancy than street drugs because of the safety standards set by the U.S. Food and Drug Administration (see Question 27), but again, using even a legal drug in amounts other than the intended dose will have unknown effects on the baby; most drug research focuses on the impacts of legal use at legitimate doses rather than excessive or illicit use. Even used at prescription levels, pain medications such as oxycodone (OxyContin), hydrocodone (Vicodan), hydromorphone (Dilaudid), and other morphine derivatives can cause withdrawal symptoms, jittery or irritable behavior, and breathing difficulties in newborns. Antidepressant medications may have similar effects, depending on how much is taken and at what point in the pregnancy they are used. Sedatives, barbiturates, and muscle relaxants generally decrease the newborn's responsiveness and may cause respiratory problems. Long-term effects of any of these drugs are not known.

How it is possible, then, that even alcoholic or drug-addicted women can have healthy babies? Alcohol, drugs, and tobacco are all clearly toxic, but using them doesn't automatically mean that the baby will be severely, or even moderately, damaged. As with other risks, the extent and nature of the harm that is done depend on many factors:

- How often the mother drinks, smokes, or uses drugs
- Her overall health and physical well-being
- Whether she uses drugs/alcohol/tobacco on a full or empty stomach
- At what stage in the pregnancy the substance use occurs (and whether it stops at any point in the pregnancy)
- Factors outside of the mother's control, such as her baby's genetic makeup

Substances associated with the absolute worst outcomes are cocaine in all of its forms, alcohol, and tobacco. Other substances may cause withdrawal in the infant and other long-term physical and behavioral dysfunctions, but those three are most often associated with severe birth defects and death.

It is best to avoid using any of these substances completely in order to reduce the risk of harming the baby. If you are unable to stop, discuss the matter with your doctor so that he or she can refer you to substance abuse treatment. Understand that you will not be in any danger of arrest or prosecution if you bring up illegal drug use to your doctor; conversations with your doctor are absolutely confidential. Your doctor should be aware of any addiction issues you have. If you're addicted, your baby probably is too, and management of the baby's withdrawal symptoms after birth is best planned in advance and supervised by hospital staff. We have seen babies who were full term and otherwise healthy die because the hospital, unaware of the addiction issue, sent the babies home with their mothers, where the babies underwent withdrawal without any medical support. *A newborn who is in withdrawal from any form of legal or illegal substance is in a life-threatening, emergency situation. The only appropriate action in this case is to get immediate medical assistance for the child.* Additional resources to help with smoking cessation and drug or alcohol abuse are listed in the Appendix.

Elizabeth's comment:

I have an acquaintance who drank and used street drugs throughout her pregnancies. All three children seemed to be normal and healthy at birth, but as they've grown up they've developed learning disabilities and attention deficit disorder. Addiction is a very tough struggle, I know, but in the end, if a drug- or alcohol-using woman doesn't at least TRY to get a handle on it when she becomes pregnant, the baby will suffer the consequences. Also, getting help with the baby's withdrawal after birth is essential—Dr. Pinette told me chilling stories about losing babies to substance withdrawal. The sad irony is that these mothers probably said nothing about their substance use because they were afraid that they'd get in trouble if their babies were addicted. Unfortunately, then the babies went untreated and died—and then the mothers most likely got exactly the trouble they were hoping to avoid AND had to live with the loss of their baby! If you have this problem, it is best to swallow your pride or fear and tell your doctor the truth.

21. Is it safe to get vaccinated during pregnancy if I'm considered high risk?

It depends mostly on why you're getting vaccinated. Vaccines for some diseases, such as influenza, are considered safe after the first trimester, but other vaccines should not be administered to pregnant women. Table 3 lists many routine and nonroutine vaccinations according to whether they're safe for pregnant women. The good news is this: If you were born and raised in the United States, you've probably already had most of the vaccinations that aren't safe, as they're given to children and are mandatory before a child can attend school. If you grew up outside of the United States, particularly in a developing nation where health care isn't standardized, you may need a blood screen to make sure that you have immunities to certain diseases, such as measles or rubella, that are harmful to a developing fetus. For the most part, the decision to vaccinate is determined by weighing the potential benefit against the risk to the fetus. Although a vaccine such as tetanus has a certain relatively low risk to the fetus, actually getting lockjaw while pregnant is a great deal worse, so giving a tetanus shot to a pregnant woman exposed to tetanus is the right thing to do. This is also true for the MMR vaccine. Generally, vaccines made with "dead" virus are generally safe and may be used if the mother has been or will be exposed to the disease. Vaccines made from a live virus pose a higher risk to the fetus and generally should be avoided unless the risk to the mother is extreme—a very rare situation. Where both types are available—as with the influenza vaccine—the inactive virus vaccine is a better choice.

22. Why does my doctor think that I may be at risk for preterm labor or other complications?

Preterm labor, like many other complications, is frequently a product of underlying health issues in the mother. Although it is generally unpredictable (many perfectly healthy women have gone into labor unexpectedly, whereas women with serious

Table 3 Vaccine Safety During Pregnancy

Disease/Vaccine	Safe During Pregnancy?	Comments
Routine Vaccines		
Hepatitis A	Probably	Actual risk to fetus has not been determined, but is probably low because it is produced from inactivated vaccine; recommended for those women at high risk of HAV exposure.
Hepatitis B	Yes	Pregnant women at risk for infection should be vaccinated.
Human Papilloma Virus	Unknown	Recommended that vaccination **not** take place during pregnancy due to lack of information about potential risk to fetus.
Influenza (inactive)	Yes	Recommended for pregnant women, after first trimester.
Influenza (live attenuated)	No	Pregnant women should be given the inactive virus vaccine in place of the live attenuated virus vaccine.
Measles	No	Most pregnant women in the U.S. will have already been vaccinated as children; immigrant women may need serum screening to determine immune status if exposed to measles.
Meningococcal (MCV4)	Unknown	Determine status if exposed to MCV4.
Mumps	No	This live virus vaccine should be avoided as mumps is known to cause problems in the fetus. Most pregnant women in the U.S. will have already been vaccinated as children; immigrant women may need serum screening to determine immune status if exposed to mumps.

Disease/Vaccine	Safe During Pregnancy?	Comments
Pneumococcal	Unknown	The safety of pneumococcal vaccine during the first trimester of pregnancy has not been evaluated, but no adverse consequences have been reported among newborns whose mothers were inadvertently vaccinated during pregnancy.
Polio	Unknown	Most U.S. women will be immune from childhood vaccination, but immigrant women may not have been vaccinated. In theory, polio vaccine should be avoided unless there is reason to believe the mother is not immune and has been exposed to polio. There is no direct evidence the polio vaccine harms fetus.
Rabies	Probably	No choice. Rabies is fatal if vaccine is not given.
Rubella	No	This vaccine contains live virus, and rubella is known to cause problems in pregnancy. It should not be administered to pregnant women.
Tetanus / Diphtheria (Td)	Yes	A pregnant woman who has not had a tetanus shot within 10 years should have a booster.
Pertussis (Tdap)	Yes	Given in conjunction with Td; the Tdap vaccine protects against pertussis and does not harm the fetus directly, but there is a risk that the baby may develop an immune response (allergy) to the Tdap vaccine, interfering with the child's immunity to pertussis. It is recommended to use Td instead of Tdap for tetanus protection unless there is reason to believe the mother is at risk for exposure to pertussis.
Varicella (chickenpox)	Unknown	Recommended that vaccination **not** take place during pregnancy due to lack of information about potential risk to fetus.

(continued)

Table 3   Continued

Disease/Vaccine	Safe During Pregnancy?	Comments
Nonroutine Vaccines (Travel/Other)		
Anthrax	Unknown	No studies have been published regarding use of anthrax vaccine among pregnant women. Pregnant women should be vaccinated against anthrax only if the potential benefits of vaccination outweigh the potential risks to the fetus.
Bacille Calmette-Guérin	Unknown	Although no harmful effects to the fetus have been associated with BCG vaccine, its use is not recommended during pregnancy.
Rabies	Yes	Because rabies, left untreated, is a deadly illness, and there is no indication that fetal abnormalities have been associated with rabies vaccination, a pregnant woman exposed to rabies should be vaccinated. If the risk of exposure to rabies is substantial, preexposure prophylaxis might also be considered pregnancy.
Typhoid	Unknown	No studies have been published regarding use of typhoid vaccine among pregnant women. Pregnant women should be vaccinated against typhoid only if the potential benefits of vaccination outweigh the potential risks to the fetus.
Yellow Fever	Unknown	The safety of yellow fever vaccination during pregnancy has not been established, and the vaccine should be administered only if travel to an endemic area is unavoidable and if an increased risk for exposure exists.
Zoster (Shingles)	Unknown	Recommended that vaccination **not** take place during pregnancy due to lack of information about potential risk to fetus.

SOURCE: Adapted from *Guidelines for Vaccinating Pregnant Women*, Centers for Disease Control and Prevention. Updated May 2007. Available online at www.cdc.gov/vaccines/pubs/preg-guide.htm (accessed September 15, 2007)

health issues have had full-term babies), certain factors can point to an increased risk of this complication. Preterm labor is more common in women in the following circumstances:

- Very old or very young mothers, especially in a first pregnancy
- An eating disorder or poor nutrition before or during pregnancy
- Smoking, drinking alcohol, or abusing drugs/prescription medications during the pregnancy
- A history of a chronic disease such as diabetes or hypertension
- An infection of the uterus or cervix during pregnancy
- Preterm labor in a previous pregnancy (the single biggest risk factor, at 30% to 40%)
- An abnormality in the cervix or uterus
- A pregnancy involving twins or multiples

Although any of these situations can point to an increased likelihood of preterm labor, the last three put a mother at greatest risk for premature birth; however, only 30% of mothers considered to be at high risk for preterm delivery actually do deliver early, while 70% of preterm deliveries are associated with no risk factors at all.

Often, this and other complications arise when multiple factors are at play, and many of the same factors that predispose a pregnant woman to preterm labor also predispose her to other complications. Several of the factors listed for preterm labor could easily be used to describe heightened risk of pregnancy complications such as pregnancy-induced hypertension (PIH), gestational diabetes, and so on. Thus, if you have any or several of these factors, your doctor will consider you to be at risk for preterm labor along with other types of complications. More information about preterm labor and many other complications is in Part Five: Complications Arising in Pregnancy.

23. What is "incompetent cervix," and how might it affect my pregnancy? How do I know whether I have this condition?

In this condition, the mother's cervix is not strong enough to withstand the increasing pressure of the growing fetus, so it opens before the fetus reaches full term. Because this condition happens without labor or contractions, it can occur without warning and generally results in either a miscarriage or a severely premature birth. No more than 1% to 2% of pregnancies are affected by this situation, but nearly a quarter (25%) of late miscarriages—that is, those occurring in the second trimester—happen because of incompetent cervix.

Because it is a relatively uncommon situation, most obstetricians do not routinely check for signs of incompetent cervix during pregnancy, so unfortunately, most diagnoses of this condition occur because the mother either miscarries or delivers prematurely. In some cases, however, certain factors may alert the physician to the potential for incompetent cervix:

- A prior history of a difficult birth that could have caused cervical damage
- A prior history of surgery or trauma to the cervix
- A malformed cervix or uterus
- DES (diethylstilbestrol) exposure (see Box)

What is DES, and how do I know if I was exposed?

Diethylstilbestrol, or DES, is a synthetic estrogen that was used between 1938 and 1971 to prevent miscarriages or premature deliveries. Although it appeared to be safe and effective for both mother and baby, its use was halted in 1971 when the Food and Drug Administration determined that it was related to a rare form of vaginal cancer in women whose mothers had been treated with the drug. Since that time, other health problems related to DES use have been found:

- In women who took DES, there is a slight increase in the risk of breast cancer.

- In daughters born to women who took DES during the pregnancy, there is an increased risk for clear cell adenocarcinoma of the vagina and cervix, reproductive tract structural differences, pregnancy complications, and infertility.
- In sons born to women who took DES during pregnancy, there is an increased risk of benign epididymal cysts.

If you were born before 1972 and your mother had at least one miscarriage or premature birth before your own birth, there is a chance that you were exposed to DES. Ask your mother whether she was given DES; if she can't recall, ask whether she had any history, either miscarriage or premature birth, that might have led to DES being prescribed. If she is no longer living or is incapacitated, ask your father or other relatives whether they are aware of any history of premature birth or miscarriage. If your mother did not miscarry at least once before your birth, it is unlikely she would have been given DES while pregnant with you.

24. If I've previously had a miscarriage or a complication, does that increase my risk of the same thing happening again?

Yes . . . and no. If you have had a prior miscarriage, you are *considered to be* at higher risk of having another. This is because some conditions that can lead to miscarriage may not change from one pregnancy to the next—incompetent cervix, as discussed in Questions 23 and 79, is a prime example. However, and this may seem contradictory, you probably are not *in fact* at any greater risk than anyone else. Miscarriages happen for many reasons, and there's no reason to think that a single miscarriage, even of a first pregnancy, necessarily indicates that you will always miscarry. Many women who have children have experienced at least one miscarriage, and studies have shown that half of these miscarriages stemmed from a significant genetic error present in the fetus. Although saying so may seem coldhearted, miscarriages are most often nature's way of removing a pregnancy that probably would not have produced a healthy child. Most of the time, the loss of the pregnancy has very little to do with the mother's health or activities. However, having multiple miscarriages—particularly one after another—is a red flag telling you and your doctor that this may not be just a spontaneous, one-time loss and that the mother may have an underlying condition that is causing the problem. In general, up to three early losses (less than 10 weeks) is considered normal. One miscarriage after 10 weeks, however, might spark an investigation because 10 weeks is when the fetal heartbeat is established—a loss of pregnancy after a heartbeat is present is very unusual.

Complications of pregnancy are a great deal trickier to predict. Some complications in one pregnancy are almost a guarantee that you'll have a similar problem with a second pregnancy. **Hemolytic disease of the newborn**, for example, may recur and be more severe in an Rh-positive child of an Rh-negative mother if she has already given birth to a child that had this disorder (see Questions 33–35). In other cases, having a particular complication increases your risk of having it again, but it's not entirely certain either way. Mothers who experienced **gestational diabetes** in one pregnancy, for instance, are at an increased risk of having it in subsequent pregnancies, but that doesn't mean that they will for certain (see Question 50). For the most part, because these complications have occurred in the past, your obstetrician will be on the lookout for them again.

25. Do chronic conditions such as diabetes, hypothyroidism or hyperthyroidism, and Cushing's syndrome affect pregnancy? Is it safe to continue my medication while pregnant? Will the dose change?

These conditions, along with a number of others, are all **endocrine** disorders—that is, they affect the hormonal balance of your body such that your body metabolism isn't functioning correctly. In diabetes, the body fails to produce enough **insulin**,

Hemolytic disease of the newborn

A condition in which the mother's immune system attacks the fetal red blood cells because of different Rh factors in their blood.

Gestational diabetes

Diabetes that occurs directly as a result of pregnancy.

Endocrine

Hormone-related.

Insulin

A hormone produced by the pancreas that processes glucose.

which is responsible for processing glucose (sugar) in the blood to provide energy to the body's tissues. This condition is extremely serious even when you're not pregnant because you must balance your insulin levels with your intake of carbohydrates—too much insulin leaves you without sufficient blood sugar to provide energy, but too little leaves you with excess glucose in your blood and could lead to other complications. Hypothyroid disease is a condition in which thyroxine, a hormone produced in the thyroid gland, is either produced in lower than normal amounts or not at all. The thyroid regulates most metabolic processes in the body, so having too little thyroxine can affect your heart rate, lower your energy levels, cause weight gain and muscle fatigue, and generally make you feel weak and run down. As you might expect, the opposite problem, hyperthyroid disorder—in which the thyroid gland produces too much thyroxine—causes different symptoms: an increased heart rate and blood pressure, shakiness, nervousness or anxiety, and weight loss. In Cushing's syndrome, an adrenal gland hormone called **cortisol** is released in excess of normal amounts, causing weight gain, easy bruising, mood swings and emotional disturbances, and abnormal hair growth on the face. Although it is very unusual for a woman with Cushing's to become pregnant—it usually renders women infertile—it does happen occasionally and is a very high-risk situation for the fetus.

Cortisol
An adrenal gland hormone.

There are many other conditions or illnesses in which too much or too little of a particular hormone is produced, but the overall circumstance in pregnancy is similar in all of them. When too much of any hormone is produced, the imbalance is likely to increase during pregnancy because the body's response to conception is *more! more!* to meet the needs of the fetus—in other words, the body fails to recognize that it has enough already. Similarly, a condition in which not enough hormone is produced will likely worsen with pregnancy because the body cannot produce more, even as the addition of a fetus to the equation means it needs more.

If you were diagnosed with an endocrine insufficiency disorder such as diabetes or hypothyroidism before becoming pregnant and were treated with medication rather than an intervention such as dietary management and exercise (commonly used in controlling mild type 2 diabetes), you will usually be told to continue taking that medication during your pregnancy. For such disorders, the medication that you're taking is likely nothing more than a synthetic version of the missing hormone. Medications such as Synthroid (levothyroxine) and Humulin (insulin) are chemically the same as what your own body would produce, and thus, it is not necessary to stop taking them—your growing fetus won't know the difference. In fact, your doctor will likely increase your dose to account for the needs of the baby. Women with diabetes who were managing the disease by diet and exercise may need to start using insulin, depending on how their blood glucose levels change in the early phases of the pregnancy.

When the disorder is characterized by overproduction of a particular hormone, management might be trickier. In hyperthyroidism, for example, medications used to treat the disorder include beta blockers, radioactive iodine, and methimazole, any of which can affect the fetus to varying severities; your obstetrician or maternal/fetal specialist and endocrinologist will need to decide how to manage the disorder in tandem. You may need to switch to a different form of treatment during the pregnancy or to reduce the level of medication you've been taking. Very close monitoring of the pregnancy will also be necessary; Cushing's syndrome, for example, has a very poor prognosis for the fetus if it is not carefully monitored, but a number of case reports show that it is possible for a woman with Cushing's to give birth to a healthy, normal baby when monitored closely.

In either case, your obstetrician and endocrinologist will keep a close eye on the hormone levels in your blood and on the growth and development of the fetus, thus making sure that he or she is not suffering ill effects from treatment of the disorder.

26. How do autoimmune diseases such as lupus, rheumatoid arthritis, myasthenia gravis, or multiple sclerosis affect pregnancy?

In an **autoimmune disorder**, the cells in the bloodstream that fight disease or repair injury have mistaken some of the body's own tissues as foreign invaders and start attacking them. Generally, such diseases are considerably more common in women than men, and some of them occur most often in the peak reproductive years. Lupus or systemic lupus erythematosus (SLE), rheumatoid arthritis, myasthenia gravis, and immune thrombocytopenia purpura (ITP) are known to occur in women of childbearing age and often occur in pregnant women. These diseases may go through periods of higher or lower activity, referred to as "crisis" or "remission," respectively, and the status of the disease at the time of conception and throughout the pregnancy is of crucial importance to the welfare of the fetus throughout its gestation.

Autoimmune disorder

A disorder in which the immune system attacks the body's own cells.

Because overactive immune cells cause the problem, the standard treatment for nonpregnant women is usually **immune suppression** (that is, treatment with drugs designed to decrease the amount or activity of immune system cells) and sometimes corticosteroids, which reduce inflammation; however, pregnancy alters the equation considerably. For one thing, a pregnant woman is naturally immunosuppressed; further immunosuppression could leave her vulnerable to serious infections (see Question 29). Even so, failure to rein in the immune system during pregnancy in some autoimmune diseases could also have dangerous effects on either mother or baby. In SLE, for example, the mother's condition generally doesn't change when she becomes pregnant, but the risks to the fetus include miscarriage or premature delivery, premature rupture of membranes, pregnancy-induced hypertension, intrauterine growth restriction, or stillbirth. Other diseases, such as rheumatoid arthritis and myasthenia gravis, may actually go into **remission** during pregnancy. Thus, caring for a pregnant woman with an autoimmune disorder is a balancing act in

Immune suppression

Treatment to decrease immune system activity.

Remission

Temporary cessation of disease.

which the physician(s) must maintain her immune system at a level that is suppressed enough that immune cells won't continue or increase their attacks on her own body's tissues, while guarding against oversuppression that would leave her open to infections. Medications used to treat such disorders may need to be changed during pregnancy, as some types of medications are harmful to the fetus (see Question 27). Above all, very close monitoring of the fetus is important. The same antibodies that cause autoimmune disease in the mother can cross the placenta and affect the fetus. Fortunately, the effects in the fetus are usually short term, but the pediatrician must be aware that the problem exists so that the baby can be treated appropriately.

Testing during pregnancy in a mother with an autoimmune disorder may include the following:

- Blood tests for specific antibodies that help track the severity of the disease
- Monitoring for signs of crisis in diseases such as SLE or myasthenia gravis
- Ultrasound monitoring of the baby's internal organs, blood flow, and overall fetal growth and development
- Fetal heart monitoring for signs of distress

Some conditions also mean that delivery will be more difficult; rheumatoid arthritis, which affects the joints, and myasthenia gravis, which affects the muscles and nerves, are particularly problematic because they can affect the mother's ability to push the infant through the birth canal. In such cases, the condition of the fetus along with the current status of the mother's disease will likely determine whether the obstetrician recommends a cesarean to reduce the impact on both mother and baby.

MULTIPLE SCLEROSIS

Multiple sclerosis (MS), an autoimmune disorder of the central nervous system, most commonly occurs in women of reproductive age. Because the disease interferes with the ability of the brain to communicate with various body systems via the nerves, it can affect all major bodily functions. It is a slowly progressive disorder characterized by periods of remission and exacerbation ("attacks"), so its impact on pregnancy depends on how far the disease has progressed at the time the woman becomes pregnant.

The good news is that multiple sclerosis does not directly affect the baby's development in the womb. Also, pregnancy does not cause the MS to progress or trigger MS attacks. In fact, women with MS will often experience remission during pregnancy, possibly related to the immune-suppression factors that occur in pregnancy. With MS, the one concern is that certain drugs used to treat may have safety issues for the fetus. However, as we note in Question 27, use of medications during pregnancy is not an all-or-nothing proposition. In some situations, even supposedly "unsafe" drugs may be used during pregnancy if the benefits outweigh the potential risks.

Complications to pregnancy are related to MS only insofar as the mother's overall physical limitations might affect her ability to carry—and more importantly, deliver—the baby. A woman with mild MS has no greater risk of pregnancy complications than any other woman. When MS has progressed to more severe effects, however, there may be greater cause for concern. For example, if the mother is wheelchair bound because of her MS, the increased pressure on her lower limbs from the growing fetus could affect blood flow to her feet and legs and, more importantly, could lead to the formation of clots that can move to the lungs—a potentially life-threatening complication for *both* mother and baby. The mother may need to take blood thinners to prevent this complication. Some women with MS have decreased lower-body sensation or even paralysis, leaving them less able to detect the onset of contractions. In such cases, the obstetrician and/or neurologist will likely monitor the mother closely for signs of impending labor during the later stages of the pregnancy.

27. Are the drugs used to treat my chronic illness safe for my baby? Should I stop taking them? Are any alternative medications safer?

We can name any number of chronic illnesses ranging in severity from mild annoyances to potentially life threatening: asthma, epilepsy, psoriasis, Crohn's disease, gastroesophageal reflux disease, eczema, and all of the autoimmune disorders in Question 26—the list seems endless. Most of these and others not mentioned are treated with medications, which often have significant side effects. So it is an obvious question: Should you keep taking medications needed to maintain your comfort and/or physical well-being? It's particularly difficult to know what's safe and what's not when virtually all medications come with a label advising you to ask your doctor before taking the medication if you're pregnant.

Medication safety is determined by the U.S. Food and Drug Administration (FDA), which oversees the research, development, and marketing of all medications that can be sold in the United States. The FDA maintains a set of categories for labeling the use of a drug in pregnancy, as shown in Table 4. However, even the FDA itself considers these categories less than perfect and prone to misinterpretation, noting:

> While this category system is a start, it's confusing and leads to oversimplification. People falsely assume that drugs labeled as category X pose the most risk in pregnancy, and drugs labeled as A pose the least. But X reflects a benefit-risk judgment, and drugs in that category may be no more toxic than drugs called C or D. Some drugs, such as oral contraceptives, land in Category X simply because there is no reason to use them in pregnancy. And a drug can fall

into Category C because there is some medium level of risk based on animal studies, or because no animal studies have been conducted. (www.fda.gov/fdac/features/2001/301_preg.html, accessed November 21, 2007)

Some chronic illnesses—asthma, diabetes, and epilepsy, among others—cause injury, serious disability, or death if the illness is not properly controlled. In such cases, even medications in categories C and D should be continued under a doctor's supervision because the benefit to the mother (and indirectly, the fetus) greatly outweighs the relatively small risk. In some maternal illnesses (asthma and diabetes, for example), the

Table 4   Current FDA Categorization of Drug Risks to the Fetus

Category	Description
Category A	Adequate, well-controlled studies in pregnant women have not shown an increased risk of fetal abnormalities.
Category B	Animal studies have revealed no evidence of harm to the fetus, however, there are no adequate and well-controlled studies in pregnant women. *OR* Animal studies have shown an adverse effect, but adequate and well-controlled studies in pregnant women have failed to demonstrate a risk to the fetus.
Category C	Animal studies have shown an adverse effect and there are no adequate and well-controlled studies in pregnant women. *OR* No animal studies have been conducted and there are no adequate and well-controlled studies in pregnant women.
Category D	Studies, adequate well-controlled or observational, in pregnant women have demonstrated a risk to the fetus. However, the benefits of therapy may outweigh the potential risk.
Category X	Studies, adequate well-controlled or observational, in animals or pregnant women have demonstrated positive evidence of fetal abnormalities. The use of the product is contraindicated in women who are or may become pregnant.

SOURCE: The U.S. Food and Drug Administration (Accessed November 21, 2007 at http://www.fda.gov/fdac/features/2001/301_preg.html#categories).

effects of uncontrolled disease can sometimes do greater harm to fetal health than a supposedly harmful medication! For other illnesses, such as eczema and psoriasis, a lack of treatment might not be potentially fatal, but can still be extremely uncomfortable, even debilitating. In such cases, the severity of the disease can be weighed against the potential risks of the medication on a case-by-case basis.

With a few exceptions, there is very little to fear from most medications, even those that have warnings on the label about the potential for birth defects. The birth defect risk of most medications is generally somewhat overrated. Very few drugs actually cause birth defects at even a modest rate. Even one drug renowned for its contribution to birth defects, the acne drug Accutane, causes birth defects at a rate of 50%—high enough that physicians advise women to take serious precautions against becoming pregnant if they're taking it, but not high enough to be considered a guarantee that an inadvertent exposure to the drug during pregnancy *will* cause serious birth defects.

The problem in ascertaining risk posed by a particular drug is that birth defects are fairly common. The natural birth defect rate is approximately 1 in 30. So if 100 women take prednisone, for example, it is statistically assured that 3 will have babies with birth defects no matter what—the birth defect would have happened anyway, prednisone or no prednisone. We only come to the conclusion that prednisone may cause birth defects if 5, not 3, of those 100 pregnant women taking prednisone have birth defects. This incidence could mean that the drug causes the additional two incidences of birth defects; however, *which* two were caused by the drug versus the three that would have happened anyway? What sort of interactions between the drug and those two additional pregnancies led to a situation in which abnormalities occurred when 98 other women didn't experience that problem? Is there some underlying, unknown circumstance in those two women that may have been triggered by adding prednisone into the mix? We have, unfortunately, too little information to answer such questions.

Thus, for women who have a chronic disease, the best advice is to sit down with your doctor to discuss any medications you are taking. Be sure that you understand completely the potential consequences of halting or changing medications that you've been on for a while, particularly if they address potentially life-threatening conditions. Changes in dose or in the type of medication may or may not be called for, but the sooner this situation is settled, the more at ease you will be in taking the medication.

28. As a cancer survivor, can I be sure that my cancer won't recur while I'm pregnant? What do I do if it does?

Pregnancy and cancer don't often coincide, but it's not unheard of, particularly with the recent trend of older women having babies. Although cancer treatment can render women incapable of pregnancy, advances in treatment and prevention of infertility related to chemotherapy or radiation therapy have allowed more women to become pregnant after cancer treatment. This is unquestionably a mixed blessing: On the one hand, women who had not had children prior to cancer diagnosis and treatment now have a greater opportunity to become mothers; on the other, these women (and their partners) must live with the worry that their cancer could recur and threaten both them and their unborn offspring. It is particularly difficult to contemplate recurrent cancer during pregnancy when the hormonal changes of pregnancy could possibly *accelerate* cancer growth, as is the case with certain estrogen-dependent breast and ovarian cancers.

As a cancer patient, you were probably advised to wait at least 2 years before attempting to become pregnant. You may even have been advised not to attempt to get pregnant at all, as most forms of chemotherapy target fast-growing, rapidly dividing cells indiscriminately, taking out the good (fingernails, hair, mucous membranes, and bone marrow) along with the bad (the cancer cells). Unfortunately, fetal cells are among the type that chemotherapy agents would target as fast-growing, rapidly dividing cells, and thus, many chemotherapeutic drugs have significant effects on a fetus. Because the possibility of relapse never completely goes away, although it is greatest in the first 2 years after treatment, some doctors recommend avoiding pregnancy altogether. That's of no help to those women who have become pregnant during or shortly after cancer treatment.

Pregnancy and recurrent cancer are unquestionably difficult and very risky situations, but steps can be taken to minimize the risks. To start, make sure that both your obstetrician *and* oncologist are aware of your pregnancy as soon as possible, particularly if your treatment for cancer was recent (less than 2 years). They will need to work as a team to monitor you for cancer recurrence and to determine how to manage your pregnancy if you need repeat treatment. In some cases, it may be possible to delay treatment until after the baby is born. In others, treatment may need to be delayed until after the first trimester (so that the baby's organs will be less severely affected by radiation or chemotherapy) but can be undertaken after that stage with only limited effects on the baby. In other cases, where the cancer is particularly fast-growing or dangerous, less aggressive therapies and techniques may be chosen that will slow, rather than halt, the cancer to buy time for the fetus to develop. The particular strategy will largely depend on the type of cancer and the available treatments, as well as how far along the pregnancy has progressed before discovery of the cancer. In all three cases, however, the goal will be to limit the harm done to either you or the baby while arresting the cancer long enough for the baby to reach a point where he or she can thrive outside of the womb.

29. Are there communicable diseases or infections that can increase the risk to me or my baby while I'm pregnant?

Infectious diseases can be risky for a pregnant woman and her unborn baby in a number of ways. Some infections are risky simply because they add new stresses on an already overstressed body. Others actually do direct harm to the mother and/or the baby, either before or immediately after birth. The good news is that you should already be immune to some of the worst if you were properly vaccinated as a child (see Table 3, Question 21). The bad news is that other infections that can do serious harm are asymptomatic and almost undetectable without a blood test—which means that if you haven't already had it, you may not be able to avoid it. There are, of course, too many such diseases to discuss in this book, but we address some of the more common concerning bacterial and viral diseases and give you pointers about how to avoid them—and what to do if you *do* get sick.

COLD AND FLU VIRUSES

We've all experienced garden-variety cold and flu bugs and know what the symptoms are: stuffy or runny nose, sore throat, cough, headache, muscle aches, fatigue, and sometimes upset stomach, nausea, vomiting, diarrhea, and lack of appetite. However, these symptoms are potentially serious because of the possibility of having dehydration coupled with systemic infections. As mentioned in Question 26, when you became pregnant, your immune system was somewhat suppressed by certain pregnancy hormones. This response occurs to protect the fetus from being rejected or harmed by antibodies in your blood, which could potentially consider it "foreign" and seek to destroy it. Of course, although it protects the fetus, it also leaves you more vulnerable to bacteria, viruses, and fungi that you encounter on a daily basis. In short, you're more likely to get sick, and when you do, you don't throw off the bug quite as easily as you otherwise might have done. The illness taxes your physical resources even more and your lowered defenses provide opportunities for the virus or bacterium to expand in your body. At the same time, many of the standard over-the-counter medications to treat symptoms and at least make you more comfortable are worrisome to pregnant women because they contain ingredients that have unknown risks to the baby. So what do you do about a bad cold—or worse, the flu?

Undoubtedly, you'll suffer much less if you take steps to avoid getting sick in the first place. For this reason, pregnant women are advised to get vaccinated against influenza at the beginning of the flu season—in fact, they're considered high-priority candidates when vaccine is in short supply. So get the vaccine, either through your doctor or a health clinic that offers public vaccination, but be aware that it doesn't necessarily mean you won't get sick with flu, flu-like viruses, or bad colds. (If you're allergic to eggs, skip the flu shot. The vaccine is produced using eggs and could trigger an allergic reaction.) Besides getting vaccinated, practice good hygiene. Some suggestions for treating cold and flu symptoms are found in Question 71.

Good Hygiene Goes a Long Way

Many simple preventive strategies will go a long way in keeping you free of viral and bacterial infections.

- Wash your hands or use an antiseptic gel frequently. The most frequent mode of transmission for viruses and bacteria from one person to another is via the hands. *Never eat without washing your hands first!*
- Also, don't share food, cups, or utensils with other people, particularly children. Saliva from the other person's mouth can carry viruses or bacteria, even if you wipe it off before using the utensil or cup.
- Wear gloves or use a handkerchief or paper towel when touching doors, cabinets, light switches, or other surfaces that others, especially children, have touched.
- Disinfect common surfaces regularly with a disinfectant wipe or even old-fashioned soap and water. These include doorknobs, bathroom fixtures, light switches, computer keyboard/mouse, telephones (particularly the mouthpiece), and tabletops—anything that you touch on a regular basis.
- Teach children to cover their faces with their elbows or shoulders to avoid spreading germs when they cough or sneeze, and avoid people who have symptoms of illness (runny nose, sneezing, coughing).
- Change sheets and pillowcases weekly. This helps limit the presence of bacteria and viruses near your mouth and nose so your chance of getting infection is lower.

If there's a risk of a more serious infection such as bronchitis or pneumonia—particularly if someone else in your family is ill with a serious lung infection—alert your doctor, as he or she may want to give you a round of antibiotics to help your overburdened immune system get rid of the infection. Maintain open communication with your doctor, and take care of yourself . . . but don't worry about your baby too much. Common colds, bronchitis, flu, and even pneumonia don't generally do direct harm to a fetus, even in the early weeks of pregnancy.

STREPTOCOCCUS INFECTION

Most of us have experienced a *Streptococcus* infection as a child, with a case of "strep throat" involving white spots on the tonsils, headache, fever, and a few days off of school to recover. This form of streptococcal infection is what is known as group A strep. Although unpleasant, it isn't overtly dangerous in pregnancy. A different form of streptococcal infection, **group B strep** or GBS, is another matter: This bacterium is found in the uterus, placenta, and/or urinary tract of between 15% and 40% of all adult women. Although it is harmless to the mother, it can be transmitted to the infant during birth and on rare occasions can have very serious, even life-threatening, effects. Unlike group A strep, if GBS is in your body, you're unlikely to know it, as it does not cause symptoms in a healthy adult woman. Fortunately, most women are tested for GBS as they approach delivery so that the mother and infant can be treated during labor with intravenous antibiotics if necessary.

Group B strep

A specific form of streptococcal bacteria.

CYTOMEGALOVIRUS

Cytomegalovirus (CMV) is a virus that is generally harmless to adults and even children but can be a significant problem to an unborn fetus. Although most babies born with CMV have no health problems, it can cause congenital birth defects such as hearing loss, vision impairment, and varying degrees of mental retardation and/or coordination problems. Generally, the earlier the fetus is infected with CMV, the greater the

Cytomegalovirus (CMV)

A virus generally harmless to adults or children, but dangerous to unborn babies.

possibility and extent of birth defects. Fortunately, it is unusual for mothers to pass CMV to their unborn babies unless they are infected with CMV for the first time while pregnant—and even then, only about one third of those women actually transmit the virus to the fetus.

Because CMV usually has no symptoms in adults, it's hard to diagnose. The symptoms, when they do appear, are similar to mononucleosis: swollen glands, fever, sore throat, and fatigue. If a pregnant woman is diagnosed with a CMV infection, an amniocentesis can be done to check fetal fluids or blood for signs of infection. Also, an ultrasound can identify some physical signs that could signify possible infection, including low amniotic fluid levels, intrauterine growth restriction, and enlarged tissues in the brain. After birth, the baby's blood, saliva, and urine can also be tested for CMV. In severe situations of CMV infection, the mother can be treated with antiviral drugs such as acyclovir to reduce the extent of the infection.

CMV is transmitted by exposure to droplets of saliva or mucus—in other words, the same way the common cold is transmitted. Throughout your pregnancy, practice good personal hygiene. If you develop a mononucleosis-like illness, you should be checked for CMV infection. Your doctor can test for CMV antibodies to determine whether you have already had CMV infection.

MEASLES, MUMPS, RUBELLA, CHICKENPOX, AND FIFTH DISEASE

Measles, mumps, rubella, chickenpox, and fifth disease (parvovirus B19) can all cause serious health problems for a fetus if the mother contracts the disease while pregnant. Most women in America are immune to most of these diseases either from a vaccine or from a childhood infection—the only exception is fifth disease, for which no vaccine exists. However, 50% to 70% of adults are already immune. Unfortunately, even for those diseases in which vaccination is routine, you *still* might not be immune. For example, there have been instances in which the rubella vaccine given to a child doesn't result in long-term immunity, so an adult woman looking back at her childhood vaccination records may *think* she's immune to rubella, but she isn't. This is uncommon, but it does happen. The solution for a woman who *isn't* pregnant is to get vaccinated again in the hope of establishing lifetime immunity. This situation also exists with the recently introduced chickenpox vaccine; long-term data are not available to verify whether the vaccination is as effective in providing long-term protection as a bout of the actual disease in a child seems to be. If you haven't actually had chickenpox but were vaccinated instead, have a blood screen to verify that you are immune from chickenpox. Of course, if you haven't had chickenpox and weren't vaccinated, you definitely aren't immune.

Measles, mumps, rubella, chickenpox, and fifth disease can be very dangerous in pregnancy, as they can cause birth defects, miscarriage, stillbirth, premature delivery, or lifelong health problems in the baby. Many health care providers suggest that you get screened to verify immunity to all of these diseases before getting pregnant. That advice, however, is not helpful if you get pregnant unexpectedly. If you are already pregnant, you can have an antibody screen to make sure that you have antibodies to all five diseases. If you do, your worries end there (at least with respect to those particular infections), and if you don't, be extra cautious about avoiding those illnesses you haven't yet had. Avoiding exposure to rubella, mumps, and measles shouldn't be hard, as vaccination has made them extremely uncommon, but chickenpox and fifth disease may be difficult to avoid, particularly if you work around young children. Children are the natural hosts of chickenpox, and the now-routine use of the vaccine has not lowered their tendency to spread it—indeed, exposure to a recently vaccinated child can occasionally result in a case of chickenpox in a nonimmune person. Chickenpox in the mother can cause severe neurological problems in the fetus (rarely), but most of the time it is the mother, not the baby, that suffers most.

Chickenpox is infinitely more unpleasant if you catch it as an adult, leading to complications such as pneumonia. Fifth disease does not have a vaccine at all and is most infectious before symptoms appear—by the time you learn that a child you've had contact with is sick, you've probably already been exposed. Fifth disease can cause anemia in the fetus, which left untreated may lead to heart failure. If you are not immune and can't avoid children altogether, the best bet is to fall back on high standards of hygiene. If you have any of these diseases, your obstetrician will monitor your pregnancy closely and take appropriate action if complications occur—particularly with fifth disease, the anemia that develops in the fetus can be treated with transfusions, and weekly monitoring with ultrasound allows more direct intervention if signs of heart failure are observed.

TOXOPLASMOSIS AND LISTERIA

If you're a cat owner, you've likely already been warned against changing the cat's litter box, because cats sometimes carry an organism called *Toxoplasmosis gondii*, which can cause miscarriage or birth defects. Although the seriousness of **toxoplasmosis** infection in an unborn or newborn infant is quite real, the danger of infection from your cat's litter box has been somewhat overstated—you're actually much more likely to become infected by eating undercooked or raw foods; also, if you own an infected cat, you're probably already immune. Still, you can take certain precautions if you own cats—the urgency of these precautions is greater for owners whose cats go outdoors and potentially hunt and kill wild birds or mice (which could carry the parasite and transmit it to the cat) than for owners whose pets stay indoors and eat only processed (not raw) foods.

Toxoplasmosis

A bacterial infection carried in raw meat and occasionally found in cats.

- Ask another member of your household or a friend to change the litter box for you, or wear rubber or latex gloves when you do it. Make sure that you wash your hands thoroughly afterward. Change the box frequently—once weekly at minimum, but daily if possible.

- During your pregnancy, give up any gardening that requires digging in the soil. Even if your own cat is typically indoors, it is possible that feral cats or cats whose owners allow them to roam have been using your garden as a litter box, and you could acquire toxoplasmosis from the soil as a result.

- If kitty brings you a "gift" from the great outdoors, make someone else dispose of the carcass—wild birds and mice are often the source of toxoplasmosis infections.

Two other precautions apply to all pregnant women: (1) eliminate undercooked meats from your diet, and (2) when serving raw vegetables, wash them thoroughly in hot water before eating them. Particularly with root vegetables (carrots, potatoes, onions, etc.), make sure that they are very well cleaned and peeled, as *Toxoplasmosis* and other bacteria found in soil can cling to the exterior skin. Cold cooked meats (hot dogs, deli meat) should be cooked again and eaten hot to ensure that any bacteria are killed. Be certain that any dishes or utensils that come into contact with raw foods are thoroughly washed in hot water before using them to prepare other foods, and wash your hands with soap after handling all raw foods. Do not eat any leftover food that was not sealed and refrigerated promptly after being served. Eat all cooked meat medium-well or well-done, not rare or even medium, to ensure than any bacteria are killed.

These same techniques will also help you avoid *Listeria*, which is the reason your doctor may have instructed you to stay away from soft cheeses and lunch meat. Like *Toxoplasmosis*, *Listeria* is often present in the soil and can be carried by animals, but the primary source of **listeriosis** in pregnant women is exposure through food—specifically, uncooked (or undercooked) meats and vegetables, unpasteurized dairy products, and some packaged foods such as deli meats. Like toxoplasmosis,

Listeriosis

A bacterial infection found in raw or undercooked meats.

listeriosis can be treated with antibiotics, but both diseases can be dangerous to the fetus unless treated promptly. Symptoms resemble a mild flu (muscle aches, nausea, vomiting, and so on); therefore, contact your doctor if you feel as though you have the flu, particularly if you have recently eaten any undercooked meat or unpasteurized dairy foods.

SEXUALLY TRANSMITTED DISEASES

At the risk of stating the obvious, pregnancy usually comes about through unprotected sex—and that could mean exposure to a **sexually transmitted disease (STD)**. Most of the commonly known STDs have significant, dangerous effects on a fetus or a newborn. STDs can be transmitted from the mother to the baby before, during, or after the baby's birth. Some (syphilis) cross the placenta and infect the baby while it is in the uterus; others (gonorrhea, chlamydia, hepatitis B, and genital herpes) are transmitted as the baby passes through the birth canal. Human immunodeficiency virus (HIV), the virus that causes AIDS, can cross the placenta during pregnancy, infect the baby during birth, or (unlike most other STDs) infect the baby through breastfeeding.

Some of the harmful effects of STDs in babies include stillbirth, low birthweight, pneumonia, neurologic damage (ranging from brain damage to lack of coordination in body movements), blindness, deafness, acute hepatitis, meningitis, chronic liver disease, and cirrhosis. Because the damage done to an affected infant can be severe, most routine prenatal care includes screening tests for STDs starting early in pregnancy and, if necessary, repeated close to delivery. Many of these infections, including HIV, can be eliminated or made less severe in the baby if the infection is treated at birth (there is no way to cure HIV in the mother at this time). In our practice, we routinely screen for HIV because we can reduce the risk of transmission of the virus to the baby from 30% to less than 1% with appropriate treatment—but that's *only* possible if we know the infection exists.

Sexually transmitted disease (STD)

Any of several diseases passed between sexual partners.

Appropriate treatment can reduce the risk of transmission of HIV to the baby from 30% to less than 1%—but that's only possible if we know the infection exists.

30. Could my past history of depression, anxiety, or eating disorders affect my pregnancy?

Depression and anxiety do not directly affect the fetus, but they can impact the pregnancy by jeopardizing the mother's general health. Women suffering from mood disorders may get poor nutrition, sleep, and health care, the lack of which could indirectly affect the fetus's health. Particularly if depression or anxiety disorders are coupled with other risk factors, the effects of the mood disorder could be serious. Even if the mood disorder is the only risk factor, it can have potentially significant effects. For example, a woman suffering from clinical depression could come down with influenza but, because of her depression, fail to get treatment for her illness. Untreated, she could become dehydrated and go into preterm labor. Although the depression did not cause the preterm labor, it clearly was an important factor predisposing the situation. Mood disorders therefore can be the indirect cause of potential harm to the fetus.

Eating disorders such as **anorexia** and **bulimia** are particularly common in young women and are therefore a risk factor for pregnancy. Such disorders stress the body and can have long-lasting effects on overall health. Even if the eating disorder is long past, the iron, calcium, and folic acid stores in the mother's body may be depleted, so she may require extra nutritional support for a healthy pregnancy. Moreover, the distorted body image that tends to accompany such disorders (where women believe themselves to be overweight or "fat" even when they are skeletally thin) may affect her understanding of her health during pregnancy. Unquestionably, pregnant women *do* look "overweight," so a woman who has previously suffered from an eating disorder may find herself obsessing over her body image as she grows larger with pregnancy, risking a relapse of her eating disorder.

Anorexia

An eating disorder in which poor body image impairs the ability to eat, leading to gradual starvation.

Bulimia

An eating disorder characterized by alternating cycles of binge eating and purging (vomiting).

If you have suffered from a mood or eating disorder in the past—particularly if you required or are still receiving medication for your condition—be sure to discuss your pregnancy with your mental health professional as early as possible. The hormonal changes of pregnancy can affect your moods in unexpected ways. Eating disorders, in particular, may have left your body susceptible to nutrition-related complications (iron-deficiency anemia, for example). In all cases, you must continue to receive treatment for such disorders (see Question 89).

31. Do fertility treatments affect my risk level for complications in the pregnancy?

Getting pregnant by means of fertility treatments almost automatically puts you in the high-risk category for two reasons. First, the need for fertility treatments usually correlates with some health circumstance that is already a risk factor: age, endocrine imbalances, or other underlying health issues in the mother. Second, the use of fertility treatments greatly increases the possibility of multiple fetuses. Particularly with some of the more advanced methods, such as in vitro fertilization, the chance for higher-level multiples (triplets, quadruplets, etc.) is considerably greater.

Because of your need for fertility treatments, you will likely have had close care from your OB/GYN, a fertility specialist, and/or any other specialists (an endocrinologist, for example) during preconception. This care is an essential in reducing your risk of complications and will likely continue throughout your pregnancy. This could mean that you will be offered additional testing or that some routine tests will be followed up more aggressively if the results are borderline. Undoubtedly, determining whether you are carrying multiples will be one of the first priorities for ultrasound examination in the first trimester.

32. How might lung diseases such as asthma, emphysema, or cystic fibrosis affect my pregnancy?

Asthma and emphysema are both obstructive lung diseases, meaning that they prevent free flow of air (and consequently oxygen) through the bronchial passages. Both asthma and emphysema show a characteristic abnormality when **pulmonary function testing** is performed. The difference between the two diseases is that the air-flow abnormality is fully reversible ("correctable") in asthma, whereas the air-flow abnormality in emphysema is "fixed" or irreversible. Emphysema (but not asthma) is also characterized by the damage of normal lung tissue, especially of the latticework that supports the alveoli. More advanced forms of emphysema will thus affect the gas-exchanging functions of the lung and interfere with the proper function of the alveoli in their role as transfer stations for oxygen going from the air to the bloodstream. Finally, the most common forms of emphysema are associated with cigarette smoking, but asthma is not, although cigarette smoke is sometimes an asthma "trigger." Although asthma is by far more common in women of childbearing age, the recent upsurge in pregnancy among women over age 40 makes it more likely that obstetricians will see pregnant women with emphysema.

Pulmonary function testing

Testing to determine how well lungs transfer oxygen into the bloodstream.

Cystic fibrosis is a genetic disease in which the lungs are clogged by thick, sticky mucous secretions. These secretions are prompted by the defective gene. The disease creates a very high risk of lung infection in people who have it, with the additional effect that it prevents the normal processes of enzyme production in the pancreas so that absorbing nutrients from food is more difficult. Recent advances in medicine have enabled children with cystic fibrosis to live beyond childhood into their 30s and 40s, and pregnancy in women with cystic fibrosis is likewise becoming more common.

In any of these disorders, uncontrolled disease limits the mother's ability to take in sufficient oxygen (with cystic fibrosis, the mother may also have difficulty gaining enough weight to support the pregnancy). Although the body does compensate somewhat for the oxygen demands of the fetus by increasing the lungs' capacity to absorb oxygen, the changes may not be sufficient to counterbalance the oxygen deprivation that can occur, particularly later in pregnancy when the uterus presses upward against the lungs, making it uncomfortable for the mother to breathe deeply. Oxygen deprivation can increase symptoms such as dizziness, fainting, nausea/vomiting, and fatigue, and mothers with poorly controlled asthma appear to be at greater risk for complications involving high blood pressure (see Questions 45–49). For the fetus, poorly controlled maternal lung disease can lead to premature birth, low birthweight, and other forms of distress (see Questions 40 and 41). Severe or sustained oxygen deprivation caused by frequent, serious episodes of breathing difficulties (the kind that require emergency care) can be disastrous to the fetus. Hypoxia affects the fetus faster and more seriously than the mother, so it must be addressed before it reaches that level of severity; in rare cases, supplemental oxygen and even intubation can be used to ensure that the mother and fetus receive adequate oxygen.

Fortunately, lung disorders such as asthma and emphysema are easily addressed and treated with inhaled medications that have very few risks to the fetus. In both diseases, keeping the lung function as normal as possible is important. If you have asthma or emphysema and are not seeing a **pulmonologist** (a doctor specializing in lung disease), it might be wise for you and your OB/GYN to consult one so that your treatment regimen can be updated if the changes of pregnancy affect your lung capacity. If you are already under the care of a pulmonologist, let him or her know that you are pregnant, and ask whether a change is needed in your asthma or emphysema management plans. You will likely be advised to continue the

Poorly controlled maternal lung disease can lead to premature birth, low birthweight, and other forms of distress.

Pulmonologist

A doctor specializing in lung disease.

strategy that you're currently using, which might combine the use of inhaled medications with lifestyle factors such as avoiding asthma triggers or limiting exposure to bronchial stressors like colds or flu, cigarette smoke, and pollution. Your pulmonologist may, however, recommend changes if your lung disease is very severe, is not well controlled, or is being controlled with oral corticosteroid medications. In the latter case, the medications should be reviewed by both the OB/GYN and pulmonologist to make sure that any effects on the fetus are limited. In most cases, the risk of harm to the fetus from the medication is far outweighed by the potential risk to both mother and child if asthma or emphysema is uncontrolled for even a short time.

Cystic fibrosis is not so easily managed. Mothers with cystic fibrosis tend to be considerably sicker than those with asthma or emphysema and are at much greater risk for premature delivery. Your pulmonologist and maternal/fetal specialist will likely monitor both your symptoms and your baby's progress very carefully throughout the pregnancy.

The most important advice in these situations is this: Keep in close touch with your doctor, and avoid anything that stresses your ability to take in oxygen. This obviously means you cannot smoke, but it also means that if you live with a smoker, he or she must not smoke in your presence or even indoors—it isn't enough to simply open a window or take it to another room because smoke, like air, travels from room to room. If your smoking roommate won't quit, he or she must smoke outdoors. Likewise, limit your likelihood of contracting a lung disease: Avoid people who are sick, practice good hygiene, get vaccinated against influenza, and stay well hydrated. Lung infections should be treated at first sign with decongestants and antibiotics, if necessary. These simple practices could mean the difference between a complicated versus an uncomplicated pregnancy.

PART FOUR

Preexisting Risks: Baby's Health

What sorts of health problems can occur in an unborn baby?

How are prenatal health problems or risks diagnosed?

Can anything be done to treat my unborn baby's health problems?

More . . .

33. What sorts of health problems can occur in an unborn baby?

Health problems in unborn babies are relatively uncommon—certainly not as common as health problems in the mother. This occurs for several reasons: First, health problems related to genetic errors and mutations most often result in miscarriage. Second, harmful substances and organisms are generally eliminated by the mother's immune system, liver, and kidneys before they can cross the placenta and affect the fetus. Nonetheless, some conditions can and do affect unborn babies.

CONGENITAL DISORDERS/ BIRTH DEFECTS

In about 1 in every 30 pregnancies, the fetus develops abnormally. Some of these abnormalities are minor—along the lines of an extra finger or toe. Others are significant, profoundly affecting the baby's mental and physical development before and after birth (for example, fetal heart disorders, a fairly common congenital disease). When such an abnormality affects the functioning of an organ, limb, or other physical entity, the baby may require surgical intervention—surgery repairing cleft lip and palate, for instance. In cases of heart disorders, some forms of spina bifida, or **gastroschisis** (a hole in the abdominal wall that causes part of the intestines to spill out into the amniotic sac), surgery may be required immediately after or even before the baby is born (see Question 35), although sometimes, even with cardiac problems, the disorder may resolve itself. Other congenital disorders are so severe that the baby's chances for survival are limited; some of the genetic diseases described in Question 38 fall into this category, as does the neural tube defect anencephaly.

Gastroschisis

A condition in the fetus in which a hole in the abdominal wall causes part of the intestines to spill out into the amniotic sac.

INFECTIONS TRANSMITTED FROM THE MOTHER

A number of illnesses can pass through the placenta to infect the fetus, as described in Question 29. Some of these, such as cytomegalovirus, can be fatal to an infant because a newborn's immune system is incapable of containing the infection. Others, if acquired early enough in the pregnancy, can lead to birth defects by interrupting the correct development of one or several organ systems; chickenpox in a pregnant mother, for example, can cause eye problems, poor growth, small head size, delayed development, and/or mental retardation in the fetus. Alternatively, an infection can create health problems in an otherwise healthy fetus. Fifth disease, for instance, can cause anemia in a fetus that may be fatal if left untreated.

TUMORS

In very rare circumstances, routine ultrasound screening detects an abnormal mass that turns out to be a tumor, usually a benign (noncancerous) growth. Although the tumor is benign, it can still be potentially life threatening to the fetus if it grows very large or affects crucial organs. Prognosis for a fetus diagnosed with a tumor depends on the tumor location: Certain tumors have a high survival rate (abdominal tumors, for instance), whereas others, especially brain tumors, do not. Fetal tumors can sometimes be treated before birth using different techniques: Cystic tumors may be surgically punctured and drained, whereas solid tumors can be surgically excised or treated with radiofrequency ablation to cut off blood supply to the tumor, hindering the tumor's growth so that the fetus can survive to delivery, at which point the tumor is removed. Such treatments are performed only at specialized centers, however, and some techniques are still experimental. Fortunately, fetal tumors are very rare.

BLOOD FLOW AND COMPATIBILITY DISORDERS

Certain common health problems develop from insufficient or excessive blood flow through the placenta or the umbilical cord. These include umbilical cord complications (Question 44), placental abruption (Question 43), and blood flow restriction related to elevated blood pressure, as occurs in pregnancy-induced hypertension, HELLP syndrome (Question 47), and similar situations (Questions 45–49).

A somewhat different blood disorder that can affect unborn babies is called hemolytic disease, of which Rh disease is the most commonly known example. This disorder occurs when the mother and baby each have a different Rh factor in their blood (most often in an Rh-negative mother and an Rh-positive baby). The mother's immune system recognizes the baby's Rh factor as foreign and develops antibodies to the baby's blood type. In a first pregnancy, this usually does not cause any problems or complications but can cause trouble in any subsequent pregnancies. In those situations, the mother's immune system is mobilized against the fetus's red blood cells. The fetus becomes anemic, and its body attempts to compensate by producing red cells faster than normal. As the anemia progresses, the liver, spleen, and heart become enlarged, and fluid builds up in the fetal tissues and organs, sometimes leading to heart failure. Prevention of Rh disease involves using RhoGAM, a synthetic immune globulin that reduces the ability of the mother's immune system to react to her baby's cells. The baby is also monitored by ultrasound to detect signs of anemia and heart failure and is either delivered early or given in utero blood transfusions until he or she is mature enough for delivery.

MULTIPLES

Some complications occur in only multiple pregnancies. For example, **twin transfusion syndrome** develops with identical twins that share a placenta. Blood vessels connect within the placenta and divert blood from one fetus to the other, causing one twin to become anemic, while the other has excess blood in its veins. If this occurs early in pregnancy, it is almost always fatal to one or both of the twins if not treated; later in pregnancy (after about 30 weeks), it is possible to deliver the twins and care for them in the NICU. Treatment using lasers to disrupt blood vessels is often successful, as is drawing excess fluid from the twin with too much blood to help balance the pressure on each twin's vessels.

Twin transfusion syndrome

A condition in which identical twins that share a placenta have unequal amounts of blood in their bodies.

A very rare but well-known complication affecting multiples is **conjoined twins**, frequently called "Siamese twins" in reference to the nineteenth-century conjoined twins Chang and Eng, who were from Siam and were made famous by P. T. Barnum as a circus oddity. Although conjoined twins can be detected by ultrasound, few treatment options are available, particularly if the twins share vital organs (and most do). Approximately half of conjoined twins are stillborn, and a portion of those born alive have other congenital abnormalities that make survival impossible, even were they to be separated. Of the remainder, only about 25% of conjoined twins born alive survive more than 24 hours, and separation of the twins is often a risky, complicated endeavor that can mean the death of one or both twins. If performed, it is usually not undertaken until the twins are old enough to ensure that their overall health is stable.

Conjoined twins

Twins that fail to separate during development of the embryos.

34. How are prenatal health problems or risks diagnosed?

Most prenatal health problems are diagnosed through use of the screening tests described in Question 11. The routine blood tests that check maternal and fetal hormone levels, antibodies, and blood cell counts, the urinalyses that screen for the presence of glucose and protein, and the weight and blood pressure readings taken at each visit generally are the first indicators of problems in the pregnancy. Unfortunately, these tests are not always able to pinpoint whether the problem is with the mother's health or the baby's, although they can sometimes suggest potential diagnoses. Abnormalities in these routine tests will generally lead to more extensive testing to both rule out some potential problems and zero in on a diagnosis. When the baby has a potential health issue, an ultrasound examination of the fetus and placenta is usually taken. An ultrasound can answer a lot of questions about the fetus's health by verifying the functioning of the fetus's organs, whether the fetus is growing and moving as expected, the amount of amniotic fluid present in the amniotic sac, and the quality of the blood flow between the placenta and the fetus. Many diagnoses can be made based on blood/urine results coupled with ultrasound observations, but ultrasound is not capable of definitively diagnosing all problems, particularly specific genetic disorders or blood disorders such as hemolytic disease or fetal anemia. For those diagnoses, invasive tests such as amniocentesis, CVS, fetal blood sampling, and placental biopsy are used to examine the fetus's blood or DNA and determine whether there is an identifiable problem.

Not all fetal disorders are diagnosed before birth.

Many fetal disorders can be diagnosed prenatally, although not all fetal disorders are. A health problem with the fetus can commonly be discovered only at birth or even afterward, during the child's first months or years. Even if your doctor has highly skilled pathologists and ultrasonographers, sometimes symptoms of the disorder just don't show up in the tests and screenings performed throughout the pregnancy. The opposite is also true: An apparent complication may turn out to be a misreading of the available data. Parents are sometimes given a scary diagnosis, only to learn later that in fact their child is fine. No screening test is perfect, and the results are only as good as the person interpreting them; therefore, it is very important that any diagnosis be confirmed at a center with highly skilled personnel. Do not hesitate to ask for a referral for a second opinion, and indeed, many specialists will encourage you to get one—not out of fear of being wrong, but because they want you to be secure with the diagnosis before considering complex and risky treatment options.

35. Can anything be done to treat my unborn baby's health problems?

Very often, the "treatment" of a specific health problem involves monitoring the fetus closely to ensure that it is not in distress, but otherwise, allowing nature to take its course until the fetus is at full term (or nearly full term). This happens because intervention in the pregnancy is sometimes not necessary and indeed is counterproductive. In general, larger babies are more likely to thrive outside the womb than smaller babies. Therefore, unless the fetus is in imminent danger, the uterus is the safest place, as long as nutrients and oxygen are reaching the fetus. Bringing the child into a world full of physiological stresses and disease-causing organisms cannot help matters.

For this reason, health care providers prefer to wait until the mother spontaneously delivers a full-term baby before providing surgery, medication, or both. The exception is when the fetus's situation in the uterus is potentially dangerous. For example, if the fetus is receiving inadequate blood flow (for example, from placental abruption), immediate delivery would be required, either through cesarean section or by induction of labor and care in a NICU. If the situation permits, the health care team may give corticosteroid medications in the week before inducing labor or performing the cesarean section to encourage lung development in the fetus (see Question 82).

Under very unusual circumstances, it is possible to provide treatment in utero. Certain congenital abnormalities can be corrected surgically even before the baby is born, but because it is a very difficult, risky procedure that requires highly skilled and experienced staff, it is usually reserved for situations when the fetus is not expected to live to full term, or even long enough to be delivered for surgery immediately after birth. A disorder called **congenital diaphragmatic hernia**, in which the liver is located in the chest, causing the lungs to be compressed and poorly developed, may call for fetal surgery to lessen the severity of the problem and permit the baby to live to birth, at which point it will undergo further corrective surgery. Most babies with this condition, however, still do better being carried to term, with surgery performed immediately after delivery; fetal surgery is generally used only if it seems clear that a full-term pregnancy is unlikely.

Fetal surgery can be done in various ways. **Fetoscopic surgery** uses a fiber-optic scope to enter the uterus through small surgical openings so that correction of the defect can be done without major incisions and without removing the fetus from the womb. **Open fetal surgery** requires that the uterus be surgically opened as in a cesarean section, exposing the fetus so that it may be operated on. After the defect has been repaired, the fetus is returned to the uterus, and the uterus is closed again. Alternatively, if the fetus is near full term, the cesarean section might actually be performed as a means of delivering the baby, but surgery is performed on the baby before the cord is cut so that the fetus can get its oxygen from the placenta (called an **exit procedure**). This method is used when the baby has a congenital defect that blocks the airway or otherwise prevents it from breathing on its own. The umbilical cord is severed only after the defect has been corrected and the baby is capable of breathing independently or with a temporary ventilator.

36. Why are twins and multiples automatically considered a high-risk situation?

Recall from Question 1 what happens when a woman is pregnant: tremendous hormonal surges, increases in fluid retention, alteration of metabolic activity, increased strain on heart, lungs, kidneys, and so on—all in support of *one fetus*.

Congenital diaphragmatic hernia

A birth defect in which the liver is located in the chest, causing the lungs to be compressed and poorly developed.

Fetoscopic surgery

A surgical technique for operating on a fetus while in the uterus using laparoscopic methods.

Open fetal surgery

A surgical technique for operating on a fetus that involves opening up the uterus, performing surgery, and restoring the fetus to the uterus.

Exit procedure

Surgery on a fetus prior to completing a cesarean section.

Now multiply that by two for twins, three for triplets, and four for quadruplets. You get the idea. If one baby is a hefty load for even a healthy woman, then twins or multiples are an even greater burden. Of course, a woman carrying multiples may not have any complications, but obstetricians want to err on the side of caution, knowing that the burdens and risks of multiple fetuses are considerably greater. Hence, this high-risk label gets stamped on any pregnancy that involves multiples.

Some specific complications that are more common in multiple pregnancies than in singletons are as follows:

- Premature labor and birth
- Low birthweight
- Pregnancy-induced hypertension (see Questions 45 and 46)
- Placental abruption (see Question 43)
- Anemia
- Amniotic fluid abnormalities
- Gestational diabetes
- Miscarriage or "vanishing twin" syndrome (loss of one of the twins, triplets, or quadruplets; it is possible to lose one fetus while the remaining fetus or fetuses survive)

37. How can I reduce the risk of problems or complications if I'm carrying two or more babies?

The risk of complications can be reduced by taking whatever steps necessary, as discussed in Questions 8 and 10, to determine what the risks are and to prevent those that are alterable through good nutrition and healthy living. Nutrition, in particular, is of primary importance as your body seeks to support not one but two or more babies. Your doctor will recommend strategies to increase your intake of protein, calcium, iron, folic acid, and other essential nutrients to meet the needs of your fetuses. You will likely be advised to gain at least 35 to

45 pounds and to have more frequent prenatal visits (to check for complications and to monitor nutrition and weight gain). Keeping your prenatal care appointments is an important step in ensuring good health for both you and your baby!

With multiples, (1) keep a close watch for potential complications so that your obstetrician or maternal/fetal medicine specialist can intervene if necessary (see Question 35), and (2) extend the babies' stay in the uterus so that their organs, particularly the lungs, have time to mature. To prevent premature labor, the most common complication affecting multiples, you may be asked to limit your activities, reduce your workload, or leave your job far sooner than would be expected with a single baby. In extreme cases—that is, with triplets, quads, or quints—you may be put on bed rest in the second trimester, either at home or in the hospital, depending on pregnancy complications or the number of fetuses. Cervical cerclage, a technique used to prevent miscarriage or premature birth in women with incompetent cervix (see Question 79), may be used to support the cervix in containing the excess weight of multiples. If premature contractions occur, medications may be used to slow or stop them (see Question 76). Alternatively, if carrying to full term is not likely to be possible (often the case with triplets, quads, or higher), corticosteroid medications may be given to help mature the fetuses' lungs (see Question 82).

38. I have a cousin whose daughter was born with cystic fibrosis. How will I know if my own child has it? Are there other genetic diseases I should test for?

To answer this question, we need to first talk about how genetic diseases come about. At conception, when sperm meets egg in the fallopian tube (see Question 1), both are carrying 23 chromosomes in the **nucleus**—chromosomes that will form the basis of the genetic makeup of the baby that will develop after the two cells merge. The 46 chromosomes within

Keeping your prenatal care appointments is an important step in ensuring good health for both you and your baby!

Nucleus

The structure within a cell that contains the cell's genetic matter.

the blastocyst consist of 22 matched pairs plus two sex chromosomes—an "X" chromosome from the mother and either an "X" or a "Y" from the father (an XX combination produces a girl, while XY produces a boy). As the cells continually divide, these 46 chromosomes are reproduced repeatedly so that each cell has its own set exactly duplicating the original set of chromosomes in the sperm and the egg. Sometimes, however, the genes do not replicate themselves exactly, and the error(s) that creeps in becomes repeated in subsequent duplications. These errors are called mutations. Because the genetic code in a human cell is so complicated, everyone has some mutations, and most of the time they are harmless; however, some mutations are harmful, and this is where a genetic disorder or congenital problem can occur.

Four basic situations may be caused by genetic mutations:

- The mutation will have no effect on the child's health and may or may not be passed down to the child's own offspring (a **benign** mutation that is either undetectable or that has effects not relevant to health).

Benign

Causing no or little harm.

- The child can develop a congenital disorder, or birth defect, in which multiple factors working together during the division of cells in the uterus cause a significant problem in the way a fetus or child grows and develops. These factors are a combination of genetics, environmental factors, and sheer bad luck. For example, the neural tube defect spina bifida has a genetic component: a couple who has one child with this disorder is 10 times as likely to have another pregnancy affected by it. However, environmental factors can alter the risk level: The use of folic acid before and during pregnancy can lower the risk, whereas exposure to the antiseizure drug Depakote can increase it. Even in the face of both the genetic and environmental contributions, the presence of spina bifida is a toss of the dice—a matter of bad luck.

Inherited disorder

An illness or disorder caused by defects in genes passed to the child by one or both parents.

- The child may have an **inherited disorder**, in which genetic errors in one or both parents' chromosomes cause disease or damage in the child (not necessarily immediately; some inherited disorders appear only later in life). In some cases, the child need inherit a defective gene from only one parent for disease to occur (called **autosomal dominant disease**), whereas in other instances, the disease will occur only if the child gets a defective copy of the gene from each parent (**autosomal recessive disease**). An autosomal dominant disease can also occur as a new mutation, rather than being passed down from one of the parents. For this reason, many autosomal dominant genetic disorders are surprising to the parents. Some disorders, however, are "X-linked," which means that they are passed down via the X chromosome and only show up when paired with a Y chromosome—that is, when a mother passes the faulty X gene on to her son. A daughter who gets the faulty X gene from her mother does not get the disease.

- The child may be an **asymptomatic genetic carrier** of an autosomal recessive inherited disorder, which means that although that child does not get the disease, he or she has inherited a defective gene from one parent. If two people who have children together are both asymptomatic carriers, their children have a 1-in-4 chance of developing the disease, a 1-in-4 chance of having no defective genes, and a 2-in-4 chance that they will also be asymptomatic carriers of the disease.

A woman carrying a child with a genetic disorder is not automatically labeled a high-risk pregnancy. Many genetic diseases don't affect the development of the infant in the uterus, and others don't even affect the child after birth for many years, even into adulthood. Huntington's disease, for example, is an autosomal recessive genetic disorder that has no obvious effects on the child for decades after birth. Some genetic diseases, however, have the potential to cause harm to newborns or very young children, and a number of these birth defects require immediate attention after birth or, in rare cases, even before (see Questions 33 and 34).

Autosomal dominant disease

An inherited disorder in which only one defective gene is required for the disease to occur.

Autosomal recessive disease

An inherited disorder in which a defective gene from each parent is required for the disease to occur.

Asymptomatic genetic carrier

A person who, having inherited a defective gene from one parent, shows no symptoms of illness but can pass the disease to his or her children.

Congenital disorders, although very serious, are usually errors that occur during development and are only rarely inherited from parents. If someone in your family has had a child with a congenital disorder, it is extremely unlikely that you will have a child affected by the same or a similar disorder; however, for people with a known inherited disorder in their family tree (for example, cystic fibrosis), the presence of a mutation in their family tree is of considerable concern. Because cystic fibrosis develops only when a child inherits two defective genes—one from each parent—the opportunities for the disease to develop are relatively small in the overall population (fewer than 0.001% of people in the United States have this disease). When two carriers produce children, however, the risk of giving birth to a child with this disease increases to one in four (25%). The chances that someone is a carrier are still pretty slim—about 3% of the overall U.S. population carries a cystic fibrosis mutation—but the disease is damaging enough that genetic testing is routinely offered in many locations.

If this or a similar genetic disease (Table 5) exists in your family, the chances that you could be a carrier are considerably greater than average. If you're planning to have children or are already pregnant, it's worth getting a genetic test to find out if this is the case. Genetic carrier testing can be used to tell if a person carries one or more mutations of the cystic fibrosis gene and how many copies of each mutation. The test is fairly simple, using cells that are gently scraped from inside the mouth. If you are a carrier, your partner should be tested. Remember that cystic fibrosis and other autosomal recessive diseases occur only if *both* parents have a defective gene. If your partner is not a carrier, then your child or children will not have cystic fibrosis, although they could be carriers of the defective gene. If your partner is a carrier, however, performing a prenatal chromosome analysis by amniocentesis or CVS may be necessary to verify whether the baby has received two copies of the defective gene.

Table 5   Genetic Disorders That Can Be Determined Through Prenatal Genetic Testing

Disease/Disorder	Type of Testing Available	Additional Comments
Autosomal recessive genetic disorders		
Cystic fibrosis	blood screening to determine if one or both parents are carriers before birth or before conception	Testing is usually performed on an expectant mother; if she is positive, then father is tested. If both are positive, an amniocentesis can determine whether the child has two defective genes, will have CF, and will need supportive care and services. CF is the most common autosomal recessive disease; treatment advances have allowed life expectancy to extend to 30–40 years.
Tay-Sachs disease	blood screening	Testing should be considered for parents of particular ethnic groups or if family history of Tay-Sachs is present. A child with two defective genes with have Tay-Sachs, a fatal disorder for which there is no known treatment or cure. It is an uncommon disorder. Life expectancy is 3–5 years.
Sickle cell disease	blood screening	Sickle cell trait is most commonly found in people with African American and Mediterranean ancestry; an estimated 1 in 12 Americans of African descent carries the sickle-cell gene. Pre-pregnancy testing is advisable for persons with either African American or Mediterranean ethnicity. Life expectancy for a person with sickle cell anemia is ~50 years.

Disease/ Disorder	Type of Testing Available	Additional Comments
Chromosome errors		
Down syndrome (trisomy 21)	amnio or CVS	Chromosome analysis is usually only done if there is reason to believe a birth defect exist due to nuchal translucency screening results or other abnormal test results. Extra chromosome is readily apparent, but the extent to which an affected child will exhibit mental retardation and functional disabilities is generally unknown until birth or later. Life expectancy varies with severity, but average is ~49 years.
Edward syndrome (trisomy 18)	amnio or CVS	As with Down syndrome, testing is generally done only with other abnormal tests. Extra chromosome is readily apparent. Severe physical defects usually visible in ultrasound. Only 50% of pregnancies end in live birth, and of these, fewer than 10% survive past the first year.
Patau syndrome (trisomy 13)	amnio or CVS	As with Down syndrome, testing is generally done only with other abnormal tests. Extra chromosome is readily apparent. Severe physical defects usually visible in ultrasound. Of the three common trisomies, Patau syndrome is the rarest and has fewest that survive to or past birth (less than 10%).
Turner syndrome (missing X chromosome)	amnio or CVS	Chromosome analysis of amniotic cells can show the presence of Turner syndrome in 21%–67% of cases, but cannot predict how severe the disorder will be. It is rarely tested for but is sometimes found when testing for other syndromes. Always occurs in girls; a girl with Turner's often appears perfectly normal and healthy.
Klinefelter syndrome (XXY syndrome)	amnio or CVS	It is rarely tested for but is sometimes found when testing for other syndromes. Always occurs in boys; a boy with Klinefelter's often appears perfectly normal and healthy.

(continued)

Table 5   Continued

Disease/Disorder	Type of Testing Available	Additional Comments
Autosomal dominant genetic disorders		
Marfan syndrome	amnio or CVS	If one parent has Marfan syndrome, there is a 50% chance the baby will also have it. Genetic testing is therefore advisable so that treatment and prevention of complications can begin early.
Myotonic dystrophy	amnio or CVS	If one parent has myotonic dystrophy, there is a 50% chance the baby will also have it. Screening can be done if there is a known risk of this disorder. A variation of type 1 myotonic dystrophy, called congenital myotonic dystrophy, can be noted at birth. The signs and symptoms include generalized weakness, weak muscle tone (hypotonia), club foot, breathing problems, developmental delays, and mental retardation. In some cases, these medical problems are severe or life threatening.
Type I osteogenesis imperfecta	amnio or CVS	If one parent has type I osteogenesis imperfecta, there is a 50% chance the baby will also have it. Genetic analysis can sometimes predict whether a baby will be affected. Children with this condition will be susceptible to fractures and bone disorders, but it is not usually life threatening.

Aside from cystic fibrosis, a variety of genetic disorders can occur, but only some of these have an immediate impact on your child's health (Table 5). For the most part, you should undertake a test for any of these disorders only if your family has a history of them. We do *not* recommend getting tested for any genetic disorder in which the effects are not likely to occur during childhood. Huntington's disease is a prime example. Do you really want to know that your child might experience this devastating illness in 40 or 50 years, long after you're no longer able to do anything about it? When a genetic disorder exists in your family history that can profoundly affect your child as an infant or in the first few years of life, it is definitely worth investigating, particularly if there might be a need for health care or social services related to the child's potential disability (see Question 10).

PART FIVE

Complications Arising in Pregnancy

What is iron-deficiency anemia?

What is placenta previa?

What triggers preterm labor? Can preterm labor be stopped?

More . . .

39. What is iron-deficiency anemia?

Hemoglobin

A protein in red blood cells that binds oxygen from the lungs and transports it to tissues throughout the body.

Iron is a mineral that is used by the body to make **hemoglobin,** a protein in red blood cells that binds oxygen from the lungs and transports it to tissues throughout the body. When a person has insufficient iron, red blood cells cannot make hemoglobin, and oxygen is not transported effectively. This condition is called **iron-deficiency anemia.**

Iron-deficiency anemia

A condition in which a person has too little iron in his or her blood for hemoglobin to transport oxygen effectively.

Iron-deficiency anemia is fairly common, especially in women, because most people don't include enough iron-rich foods in their diets. For pregnant women, the increased oxygen and blood demands of the growing fetus can lead to anemia, even in a woman who previously has had adequate iron stores. Fully half of all pregnant women are iron deficient and are at risk for anemia, even though only about one fifth of nonpregnant women are iron deficient. Thus, obstetricians prescribe prenatal vitamins that include additional iron when a patient becomes pregnant (see Question 67); however, dietary insufficiency and pregnancy are not the only causes of iron-deficiency anemia. Other reasons for iron-deficiency can include the following:

- Intestinal disorders such Crohn's disease or celiac disease, which affect the ability of the gastrointestinal tract to absorb iron
- The use of medications called proton pump inhibitors that reduce gastric acid (generally to treat stomach ulcers), which decreases the availability of acids needed to break down dietary iron
- Gastric bypass surgery, which can limit the body's ability to absorb dietary iron
- Internal bleeding caused by uterine fibroids, hemorrhoids, colonic polyps or tumors, or regular use of aspirin, ibuprofen, or other NSAIDs
- In women, a history of heavy menstrual periods, which reduce the iron stored in the body

- A vegetarian diet that doesn't include supplemental iron, as the iron found in vegetable sources isn't absorbed as easily as iron from meat sources

In very mild cases, a person with anemia may not notice symptoms of fatigue, lightheadedness, or cold hands and feet—indeed, a pregnant woman in particular might ignore such symptoms, believing them to be related to the pregnancy. As anemia becomes more severe, other symptoms may arise, including soreness or inflammation of the tongue, brittle nails, headache, restless legs syndrome, or unusual cravings for substances other than food, such as ice or dirt (a condition called **pica**). Such symptoms should prompt an immediate call to your obstetrician.

Pica
Cravings for dirt, ice, or other nonnutritive substances while pregnant.

If you have mild iron deficiency, the baby gets his or her share of iron before you get yours; therefore, even if you're lacking a little, he or she probably has an adequate iron supply. Prolonged, severe anemia, however, puts you at risk for preterm labor or for having a low-birthweight child, and it could increase the baby's risk of being anemic as an infant. More importantly, for the mother, iron deficiency, particularly toward the end of the pregnancy, causes weakness, fatigue, decreased ability to fight infection, and rapid heart rate, which are all serious symptoms in a pregnant woman. They can be especially serious if you are in labor or have just given birth, particularly if you lose a lot of blood during childbirth. To avoid such complications of anemia, you will be prescribed a prenatal vitamin that contains iron, and you will be tested for anemia several times during the pregnancy. Testing for anemia is particularly important if, in addition to being pregnant, you have any of the other previously listed factors. Anemia is directly associated with preterm delivery, so it's one of the single most preventable factors. If you are anemic, iron supplements (or a prenatal vitamin formula with higher iron content) will be prescribed. Take your prenatal vitamin with water or orange juice, but not with milk—vitamin C in orange juice will

Anemia is directly associated with preterm delivery.

help your stomach absorb the iron, but calcium in milk can actually hinder iron absorption. Do *not* take over-the-counter iron supplements without consulting your doctor, as it *can* be poisonous if taken in high amounts!

40. What is intrauterine growth restriction? What causes it?

Small for gestational age (SGA)

See intrauterine growth restriction.

The term intrauterine growth restriction (IUGR), also called **small for gestational age (SGA)**, describes a fetus that doesn't grow at a normal rate. A diagnosis of IUGR or SGA means that the baby will have low birthweight—that is, he or she will be smaller than 90% of all newborn babies. IUGR is not the only cause of low birthweight, but it plays a part in about one third of such cases.

It may seem funny to be so concerned about a baby being small—after all, doesn't small size mean Mom will have an easier labor? Possibly, but the real problem is that when the baby's overall growth doesn't happen at a normal pace, its body tissues and organ cells may not grow as large or as numerous—a particular concern with respect to the lungs, brain, and heart, which don't function as efficiently if they are underdeveloped at birth. In short, the baby's organs might not be ready to face the outside world if they don't grow enough while the baby is in the uterus. Furthermore, if the IUGR is caused by low blood flow through the placenta, the fetus may only receive low amounts of oxygen, affecting its heart rate, potentially harming the baby before birth, or making it less able to withstand the stress of birth; however, some babies are just naturally small, so when confronted with a smaller than expected fetus, the obstetrician must determine whether the small size is just the natural condition for this particular baby or is caused by some problem. This is made by looking at the baby's overall physical condition—most particularly, whether it is proportionate and symmetrical. The doctor looks to see whether the baby's head, arms, and legs are all in the expected proportions. A baby with a normal-size head on an undersize body, or that has two leg bones of unequal length, is a baby that may be experiencing IUGR. The blood flow through the placenta is examined carefully, as insufficient oxygen and nutrients are major factors in IUGR.

Babies with IUGR may have problems at birth that include decreased oxygen levels, low Apgar scores (a series of tests after delivery that identify babies who have trouble adjusting to the outside environment), **meconium aspiration** (inhalation of stools passed in utero), difficulty breathing, hypoglycemia (low blood sugar), lower than normal body temperature, or **polycythemia** (too many red blood cells). If IUGR is especially severe, it may result in stillbirth. Some babies born with IUGR have long-term growth problems.

Meconium aspiration
Inhalation of stools passed in utero.

Polycythemia
Excess red blood cells.

Many factors can lead to IUGR, some of which are related to maternal health problems—high blood pressure, diabetes, kidney disease, anemia, heart or lung disease, malnutrition, substance abuse (including cigarette smoking), or infection. Cigarette smoking is a particularly common factor contributing to low birthweight. Other factors are related to the uterus and placenta—placenta previa or placental abruption, or other factors leading to decreased blood flow through the umbilical cord, can lead to IUGR. Finally, factors related to the fetus itself (infection, chromosome abnormalities, birth defects, and of course, multiples) may also limit fetal growth. The fetus's well-being will be investigated through nonstress tests and ultrasounds when the first signs of a problem are noticed. Depending on the stage of the pregnancy and the source of the problem, treatment may be as simple as improving the mother's nutrition, bed rest (especially with multiples), and, particularly if other risk factors are at play, early delivery.

41. What is low amniotic fluid, and why is it a problem? What can be done about it?

Low amniotic fluid, known as **oligohydramnios**, is a complication that can occur any time in a pregnancy, but it is most

Oligohydramnios
Low amniotic fluid.

common in the third trimester and is most likely to occur in women whose pregnancies are longer than 40 weeks. It is diagnosed by calculating the overall quantity of amniotic fluid as measured by ultrasound, a measurement called the Amniotic Fluid Index, or AFI.

Amniotic fluid is an essential component of fetal development. It performs three basic functions: (1) it cushions the fetus against bumps and shocks, (2) it maintains the proper temperature (for most of its time in utero, the baby has very little body fat), and (3) it fills and defines the space in which the baby's limbs and organs need to grow. Low amniotic fluid can lead to malformation of various organs or limbs and possibly to miscarriage or stillbirth, particularly if it occurs before the third trimester. Although more frequent in overdue pregnancies, low amniotic fluid can be related to a variety of other complications: placental abruption, premature rupture of membranes, birth defects, hypertension, preeclampsia, diabetes, and chronic hypoxia caused by lung disease. Sometimes, however, it is simply a product of dehydration and is resolved by having the mother drink more fluids.

Amniotic fluid is composed of a watery liquid that is produced by the mother until about 16 weeks; thereafter, the fetus also contributes by urinating. This is kind of gross, but much of what your baby is floating in is his or her own pee! This means that the level of amniotic fluid is directly reflective of how well the baby's kidneys are processing fluids and wastes and how well the placenta is functioning to send fluid and nutrients to the baby in the first place. If the placenta isn't working well, the baby will pee less because it's receiving fewer nutrients and fluids. Thus, low amniotic fluid can be a warning sign that the placenta is not well.

If the pregnancy is full term or overdue, low amniotic fluid is treated by inducing delivery. Production of amniotic fluid naturally decreases at about 40 to 42 weeks as the placenta reaches the end of its natural life; thus, the problem will only get worse if an overdue pregnancy is allowed to proceed. Low amniotic fluid can lead to labor complications (see Question 55); therefore, doctors will sometimes add fluids through a catheter during labor.

In a pregnancy that isn't full term, the cause for this problem must be determined. Most of the time, the ultrasound specialist who noted the low amniotic fluid also would have checked for signs of birth defects, placental abruption, and other potential causes. If none of these was observed, the obstetrician will likely look for "hidden" causes in the mother's health: dehydration, gestational diabetes, hypertension, and other health problems. Many times, improving the mother's hydration will solve the problem, but when it doesn't, the pregnancy is monitored carefully to make sure the fetus is not in distress. Early delivery by induction or cesarean section is an option if it is.

42. What is placenta previa? How is it diagnosed? What are the risks to mother and baby when placenta previa occurs?

As described in Question 1, the placenta acts as the gateway between the mother's and the baby's bodies through which nutrients and oxygen are passed. It develops in the spot where the embryo attaches to the wall of the uterus. Occasionally, this location is low in the uterus (next to or on top of the cervix) so that the placenta grows over the cervical opening—in other words, the placenta is located between the baby and its eventual exit. This is called placenta previa (or partial placenta previa if the cervix is incompletely blocked). Clearly, having a blocked pathway in which the baby must leave the uterus presents a fairly major problem! It is not always as bad as it sounds, however; unless the placenta is directly atop the cervical opening, completely blocking it, there is a fairly good chance that as the uterus expands with the pregnancy, the placenta will shift away from the cervix so that it no longer impedes the baby's progress into the birth canal. In fact, anywhere from 20% to 40% of all pregnancies have some form of placenta previa in the early stages—this extremely common problem usually resolves itself.

Placenta previa is diagnosed with an ultrasound. If a low-lying placenta is noted, the obstetrician will most likely periodically request additional ultrasounds through the pregnancy. If the problem resolves by itself (the most common situation), no further action is needed, but if the placenta remains next to or above the cervix as the due date approaches, the obstetrician will most likely recommend a cesarean section. If a woman goes into labor with the placenta covering the cervix, the dilation of the cervix may cause the placenta to detach from the uterine wall well before the baby is in position to pass through the birth canal. If this happens, the baby could be deprived of oxygen for what might be an extended period and could be stillborn. This situation also presents a fairly high risk to the mother, potentially leading to serious blood loss or damage to the uterus that could require a hysterectomy. Rather than risk either of these highly dangerous circumstances, a cesarean section can provide a much safer delivery.

43. What is placental abruption? What does it do to the mother and the baby?

Placental abruption is a condition in which the placenta separates from the wall of the uterus, either partially or completely, before birth. It most commonly occurs as a result of a blow to the abdomen (during a car crash, a fall, or due to domestic abuse) or as a by-product of uncontrolled hypertension in the mother. Of course, abruptions can sometimes occur for no apparent reason. Complete abruption is a life-threatening complication for both the fetus and sometimes the mother; when it is partial, it is less critical for the mother unless accompanied by hemorrhage or shock, but it can still cause significant distress or injury to the fetus depending on how much of the placenta has pulled away from the uterine wall.

Treatment of placental abruption depends on the extent of the problem and when it occurs in the pregnancy. If it happens near the due date, delivery of the baby may be the safest action, preferably by inducing labor for vaginal delivery unless there are signs that the fetus is in distress. If symptoms of abruption occur before 36 weeks and the fetus is not in distress, treatment may consist of monitoring the fetus until it is mature or signs of distress are observed, whichever comes first, before inducing labor or scheduling a cesarean. If the fetus is in distress, no matter when before or after the 36-week mark (assuming it has at least developed to the point of being viable outside the womb, generally 23 or 24 weeks), delivery by emergency cesarean followed by care in the NICU is the only alternative.

44. What are umbilical cord complications? How are they treated?

Umbilical cord complications occur when blood flow from the placenta to the fetus is inadequate. A number of situations can cause this to happen. Sometimes the cause is as simple (and devastating) as a knot in the umbilical cord that cuts off blood flow, which can sometimes occur simply as a result of the baby's movements in the uterus. Alternatively, the umbilical cord sometimes becomes wrapped around a limb or the neck. A cord around the neck, called a **nuchal cord**, is fairly common; 24% of all full-term pregnancies have at least one loop of cord around the baby's neck, and sometimes more. This is not an emergency unless the cord tightens (or has the potential to tighten during labor) around the neck to the point of strangling the baby. A cord around a limb can also be serious if the blood flow is completely cut off from the limb. If such **torsions** are discovered by ultrasound and the baby is showing signs of distress, the fetus can be delivered immediately by cesarean, but in the first, second, and early third trimester, the baby may not survive long enough to be delivered.

Nuchal cord

Umbilical cord wrapped around the neck of the fetus.

Torsions

Umbilical cord twisted around a limb or knotted around itself.

Poor blood flow can also result from an abnormality of the blood vessels in the umbilical cord. A normal umbilical cord contains 2 arteries and 1 vein, but sometimes there is only a single artery. The lack of a second artery is most often an isolated situation but can be associated with multiple birth defects in the fetus.

Cord stricture

Constriction or blockage of the umbilical cord.

Finally, **cord stricture** occurs when the umbilical cord itself is constricted or blocked. Unfortunately, this condition is not usually diagnosed or treated prenatally and almost always results in stillbirth. Cord stricture is typically found during an autopsy.

Umbilical cord complications can be detected by ultrasound. Knots, which occur in about 1% of pregnancies, are incidentally noted at birth. More frequently, however, what appears to be a knot in the ultrasound is actually a kink, which generally does no harm to the fetus. For the most part, such complications cannot be reversed or treated, and the only "therapy" available is to deliver the baby if it's in distress, usually by cesarean, thus avoiding worsening of the problem during a trip through the birth canal. An umbilical cord abnormality that severely restricts blood flow to the fetus and occurs early in pregnancy generally results in miscarriage or stillbirth, and there is rarely any way to prevent this outcome.

Pregnancy-induced hypertension (PIH)

Elevated blood pressure caused by pregnancy.

Hypertension

High blood pressure.

Systolic

Blood pressure during the exertion phase of the heartbeat.

45. What is pregnancy-induced hypertension? How is it different from ordinary hypertension?

Both **pregnancy-induced hypertension (PIH)** and ordinary, chronic hypertension have similar effects on the body—none of them good. To understand why, you need to know what **hypertension**, or high blood pressure, means. When blood pumps through the arteries and veins, it exerts pressure against the walls of these blood vessels. This pressure is not constant but changes depending on whether the heart is actively beating (the **systolic** or "top" number) or is between beats (the diastolic or "bottom" number). Blood pressure is also affected by body position (standing, sitting, or lying down), by the overall cardiovascular fitness of the individual, by the time of day, by the individual's diet, and by many other factors. When blood pressure is too high for a sustained period of time—over weeks or months, that is—it can cause damage to the blood vessels, just as high water pressure might cause a pipe or hose to spring a leak. This damage might be small and quickly repaired by platelets, but over time, repeated leaks in the same location might cause scarring that can block blood flow. Such blockages can grow to the point at which the blood vessel can no longer transport blood, potentially leading to the death of nearby tissues. People who develop severe hypertension are at risk for kidney failure, heart failure, stroke or ministroke, and damage to the eyes. In pregnant women, hypertension affects the function of the placenta by making it "age" more rapidly. The natural lifespan of the placenta is 40 weeks, after which it starts to deteriorate in much the same way an older person's heart does—and just as chronic hypertension ages the heart more rapidly, so too does PIH age the placenta. In fact, the placenta from a pregnant woman suffering from PIH looks much like heart tissue from a person 80 years or older when examined under a microscope!

Chronic hypertension represents a gradual adaptation of the body to a variety of physiological and environmental factors; it generally develops over a period of many years. Pregnancy-induced hypertension usually develops after about 20 weeks of pregnancy and progresses rapidly over the course of a few weeks. Although some increase in blood pressure is normal because of the greater fluid production in pregnancy, the increase should level off and not continue; when a consistent, continuous rise in blood pressure is observed over the course of several weeks, a diagnosis of PIH is made. Many theories exist about why it happens, but currently, no definitive answers are available about its causes, although current research suggests that it is an immune response in the mother to the "foreign" cells of her baby. Chronic hypertension, on the other

Diastolic

Blood pressure during the resting phase of the heartbeat.

Complications Arising in Pregnancy

hand, is not an immune response. One significant difference between PIH and chronic hypertension is the speed at which it progresses—PIH moves relatively quickly, whereas chronic hypertension advances slowly.

PIH is a continuum of progressively more severe symptoms. Conditions such as **preeclampsia** (also called **toxemia**), **HELLP syndrome**, and **eclampsia**, described in the questions that follow, are all hypertensive disorders that may be considered outgrowths or extensions of PIH. As with chronic hypertension, a variety of symptoms may exist, depending on the severity of the problem (see Questions 46–49), or no symptoms may be present at all. One key sign of PIH is blood pressure, measured at regular intervals, that rises steadily over the course of several weeks in either (or both) the systolic (peak) and the diastolic (resting) blood pressure readings—which are always taken while the patient is seated or standing. Normal blood pressure for a healthy, nonpregnant woman who is sitting or standing upright is generally in the range of 90/50 to 120/70 mmHg, but pregnancy can increase those readings by as much as 10 to 15 points without any cause for alarm. PIH is diagnosed only when

- Blood pressure measurements continue to steadily rise;
- Other symptoms, such as protein in the urine or hyper-reflexia, are present even without increased blood pressure;
- Blood pressure reaches 140 in the systolic and/or 90 in the diastolic measurement in a person who is seated or standing.

These readings must be consistently increasing over time—anyone can have a bad day that causes a short-term increase in blood pressure, but if high readings are part of a pattern of increasing blood pressure, it is likely PIH.

PIH is used to describe hypertension that is clearly related to pregnancy and only pregnancy; for example, a woman who

Preeclampsia

A hypertensive disorder of pregnancy.

Toxemia

See preeclampsia.

HELLP syndrome

A life-threatening hypertensive disorder of pregnancy characterized by liver dysfunction.

Eclampsia

Severe hypertension in pregnancy characterized by seizures and coma.

had existing hypertension prior to pregnancy would probably see no significant worsening of her symptoms and would continue to receive the same treatment that she'd been given before becoming pregnant; however, sometimes women with chronic hypertension develop PIH on top of their existing problem, leading to the development of more serious hypertensive crises (see Questions 47 and 48).

There is no way to prevent any of the various hypertensive disorders described in Questions 46–48, but mothers can limit the risk of a serious or life-threatening outcome for either themselves or their babies by getting regular prenatal care from a qualified obstetrician. A woman showing signs of PIH should have a monthly ultrasound screening from about 24 weeks and then weekly from 32 weeks onward.

46. What is preeclampsia?

Preeclampsia is a form of PIH in which physiological responses to increasing blood pressure have begun to occur. Symptoms such as swelling in the face, hands, and feet, protein in the urine, joint hyperreflexia (that is, exaggerated knee-jerk reflexes), blurred vision, headaches, persistent heartburn, inability to tolerate bright light, fatigue, nausea/vomiting, urinating small amounts, pain in the upper right abdomen, shortness of breath, sudden weight gain over the course of a day or two, and tendency to bruise easily are noticeable. Unfortunately, no one individual will display the same collection of symptoms as any other, so diagnosing preeclampsia is something of a guessing game. Generally, however, elevated blood pressure, urinary protein, water retention, joint hyperreflexia, and swelling are the main indicators of preeclampsia.

Elevated blood pressure, urinary protein, water retention, and swelling are the main indicators of preeclampsia.

Any woman with chronic hypertension prior to becoming pregnant would be at risk for development of preeclampsia and eclampsia. She might or might not also develop PIH. As a practical matter, however, distinguishing preeclampsia that is a product of PIH versus preeclampsia stemming from existing hypertension is meaningless—the outcome of either one is the same for the patient and the baby (see Question 49).

47. What is HELLP syndrome?

HELLP syndrome is a condition arising in women with PIH that is slightly different from standard preeclampsia, although the two are related. The acronym HELLP stands for Hemolytic anemia, Elevated Liver enzymes, and Low Platelet count, which are the important markers that distinguish this disorder. HELLP is a very serious, even life-threatening condition because it may affect liver function or cause rupture of liver blood vessels.

Women who develop HELLP are at immediate risk of preterm delivery, as progression of HELLP is a signal that the baby must be delivered for the safety of both mother and child. As a result, with a diagnosis of HELLP, corticosteroid medications are generally given to improve the fetus's lung development if the pregnancy is less than 32 weeks (see Question 82). Thereafter, the mother's condition will be monitored closely until the liver function is obviously becoming impaired, or the mother and/or fetus are too sick, at which point the baby will be delivered, prematurely if necessary (see Question 84). If the pregnancy is less than 28 weeks, some obstetricians will watch the mother for signs of crisis in an effort to prolong gestation, but this is risky because a crisis can develop in a matter of days. After the mother or the baby becomes too sick to continue the pregnancy, the baby must be delivered quickly.

48. What is eclampsia? Is it common?

Eclampsia is the most severe of the PIH hypertensive disorders. It is characterized by convulsions (seizures) and coma brought on by swelling of the brain. Fortunately, it is very uncommon, occurring in only 1 of 2,000 to 3,000 pregnancies, as most pregnant women who have any form of PIH, severe or mild, are monitored closely. An obstetrician would almost certainly recommend delivery of the baby long before the mother's condition deteriorated to eclampsia, and it is possible—although unproven—that many of the women with eclampsia are those who receive inadequate prenatal care due to poverty, limited education, or other social factors. In women who do develop eclampsia, immediate delivery of the baby is the only remedy, regardless of whether the fetus is sufficiently mature to survive in a NICU; the alternative is death for both mother and fetus. Most of the time, delivery during eclampsia is undertaken by cesarean section because vaginal delivery may take too long (more than 12 hours). Intravenous magnesium sulfate is often used to prevent seizures in pregnancies with PIH or preeclampsia during labor and the first 24 hours after delivery. This medication has side effects that include weakness, blurred vision, nausea, headaches, a sensation of being hot, and a "spaced out" feeling. Delivery usually resolves the eclampsia almost immediately, but about 2% of women and 7% of infants have complications after birth.

49. What effects do hypertensive disorders have on a mother and baby?

In pregnant women, high blood pressure (whether ordinary hypertension or PIH) often causes damage in the kidneys. High blood pressure makes the heart work harder and contributes to damage in blood vessels throughout the body. Damage to blood vessels in the kidneys prevents them from being as effective in removing wastes and excess fluids from the blood. The extra fluid in the blood vessels may then raise blood pressure even higher, damaging the kidneys still more. Of course, in pregnancy, the body is already handling excess fluids in all of the tissues, including the blood, so it strains the kidneys' ability to function from the outset. It's therefore easy to understand why high blood pressure in pregnancy is capable of spiraling upward so quickly. Luckily, the kidneys return to normal almost immediately after delivery.

In the fetus, the effects of high blood pressure can be very dangerous. The pressure of blood on the vessels in the placenta and umbilical cord damages them in much the same way as the mother's kidneys are damaged, restricting the flow of blood to the fetus. As a result, the fetus may develop intrauterine growth restriction (see Question 40). Placental abruption also is more common in such cases because the lack of blood flow in the placenta weakens the bond between the placenta and the uterine wall. Furthermore, in severe cases, the fetus may experience some of the same injuries that happen in adults with chronic hypertension: damage to the kidneys, liver, eyes, and brain. Thus, hypertension during pregnancy is a potentially very serious situation that requires close attention.

50. What is gestational diabetes? How is it different from type 1 or type 2 diabetes?

You've probably heard people complain about having "low blood sugar" when they feel tired or lack energy. The "sugar" to which they're referring is glucose, which enters the bloodstream after a meal is digested. Glucose is converted by the hormone insulin (which is secreted by the pancreas) into a form that the body's tissues can use; insulin is essential to our health because without it our muscles and other tissues don't have sufficient energy to function. **Diabetes** is a condition in which the body either does not produce enough insulin to convert the glucose into energy or does not respond properly to insulin that is present in the bloodstream (a condition called **insulin resistance**). In either case, not enough glucose gets from the bloodstream to the tissues, so the tissues are starved of energy while excess glucose remains in the blood. This situation can lead to a variety of symptoms, ranging from mildly unpleasant to life threatening, as described in Table 6.

Type 1, type 2, and gestational diabetes are the three common types. **Type 1 diabetes,** also known as "juvenile diabetes" because it most often occurs in children and young adults

Diabetes

A condition in which the body lacks the ability to produce or use insulin to convert the glucose into energy.

Insulin resistance

A condition in which the body does not respond properly to insulin in the bloodstream.

Type 1 diabetes

Diabetes occurring because insulin is not produced by the pancreas.

Table 6   Common Diabetes Symptoms

Increased thirst

Increased hunger (especially after eating)

Dry mouth

Frequent urination

Unexplained weight loss (even though you are eating and feel hungry)

Fatigue (weak, tired feeling)

Headaches

Loss of consciousness (rare)

Numbness and tingling of the hands and feet

Decreased or blurred vision

Nausea, perhaps vomiting

Slow-healing sores or cuts

Itching skin, especially in the groin or vaginal area

Abdominal pain

Deep or rapid breathing

Sweet, "fruity" breath (diabetic ketoacidosis)

Weakness or fainting spells

Rapid heartbeat, trembling, and excessive sweating

Irritability, hunger, or suddenly drowsiness (hypoglycemia)

(although it can occur at any age), is a disorder in which the immune system mistakenly attacks certain insulin-producing cells in the pancreas. Without these cells, little or no insulin is produced, and diabetes results. Type 1 diabetes most often occurs in people who have a genetic susceptibility toward it, but other factors leading to this disease are still under investigation. **Type 2 diabetes,** which is far more common in adults, occurs when the pancreas produces insulin in insufficient amounts—either because insulin resistance in the tissues means that a greater than normal amount of insulin is required to move glucose effectively or because the pancreas simply doesn't produce the expected amount of hormone. Type 2 diabetes also has a genetic component, but other risk factors such as obesity, aging, cholesterol levels, and high blood pressure are also known to contribute strongly to a person's risk of developing this form of diabetes. Unfortunately, the increase in obesity in adult women in the United States has led to a corresponding increase in diabetes.

Complications Arising in Pregnancy

Type 2 diabetes

Diabetes occurring either because the pancreas decreases its production of insulin, or the body has developed insulin resistance.

Gestational diabetes is somewhat different from either of these two types. It is an outgrowth of an imbalance of pregnancy hormones and is therefore temporary (but it does bear a relationship to type 2 diabetes). To understand how this works, you need to know a little about what happens to your blood sugar during pregnancy.

When we eat food, our blood sugar levels rise rapidly as the glucose from the meal is dispensed into the bloodstream from the digestive tract. When blood glucose reaches a certain peak level, it triggers the pancreas to release insulin into the bloodstream. This insulin converts the glucose into energy and moves it into the tissues; blood glucose levels then fall very sharply. In pregnancy, however, blood glucose levels must fall more slowly because the growing fetus also needs to collect its share of energy. For this reason, the placenta produces a hormone called human placental lactogen, which interferes with the mother's ability to use insulin properly to ensure that the mother's blood sugar level remains elevated somewhat longer than it normally would, enabling the fetus to take the glucose it needs from the mother's bloodstream via the placenta. As pregnancy progresses, something like a game of "chicken" is going on between the mother's pancreas and the placenta, as the pancreas produces ever-increasing amounts of insulin to try to compensate for the elevated blood sugar, counterbalanced by the placenta's continued production of HPL to offset the insulin and keep blood sugar levels high enough to support the fetus's rapid growth. Levels of both HPL and insulin rise during the course of pregnancy, to the point at which the mother produces insulin at roughly three times her normal, prepregnancy level.

Gestational diabetes occurs when one of two things happens: Either the body, bombarded by increasing amounts of insulin, becomes unresponsive and therefore can't process glucose as effectively as it did, or the pancreas is unable to keep up with the placenta and cannot make sufficient insulin to counteract the HPL and remove the excess glucose from the blood.

Sometimes both events occur simultaneously. Either way, the mother has constant high blood glucose levels with insufficient insulin activity, which translates to diabetes.

In a woman who was diabetic before getting pregnant, very little will change. She will still need to monitor her blood glucose and strive for good control. She may need to start using insulin if she has previously used diet and exercise alone to achieve good blood glucose control, and women who already use insulin may need to increase the dose. In either case, regular self-monitoring is important, just as it was before pregnancy. For a nondiabetic woman (or one with undetected diabetes), the diagnosis of gestational diabetes will bring on a whole new world of health issues as she learns how to monitor blood glucose levels and the importance of maintaining good control (see Question 77).

51. Will gestational diabetes affect the baby's health? Will the baby be diabetic?

Gestational diabetes can have significant effects on the baby's health if not treated promptly. One effect of gestational diabetes is that the baby is larger than usual, which makes sense because gestational diabetes allows the fetus to take in more glucose from the mother's bloodstream than is normal (Question 50). With higher blood glucose levels than normal, the baby has more "energy" available for growth, which may seem like a good thing until you realize that abnormally large size or weight can increase the risk of premature labor, problems during labor, and the need for emergency cesarean delivery. The additional glucose in baby's bloodstream has another drawback as well: The high blood glucose stimulates the baby's pancreas to secrete more insulin than it would otherwise, which can make the baby hypoglycemic after birth (when it is no longer receiving excess glucose from its mother's blood) and contributes to breathing problems. The risk of preeclampsia and stillbirth increases in diabetic mothers. Also, poorly controlled or uncontrolled gestational diabetes can predispose the baby in later life to obesity and type 2 diabetes.

52. What are the signs and symptoms of gestational diabetes? Will I remain diabetic for the rest of my life?

Unfortunately, diabetes often doesn't have noticeable symptoms. A fairly significant proportion of people who have type 2 diabetes don't have any idea that they have the disease. Furthermore, many of the symptoms of diabetes are similar to the symptoms of pregnancy—increased hunger and thirst, frequent urination, nausea, and fatigue. Thus, symptoms alone will not be enough to determine whether you have diabetes. For this reason, physicians routinely perform an **oral glucose tolerance test** (or "glucose challenge") to determine how well their patients are processing glucose. The test is typically performed between the 24th and 28th weeks of pregnancy because levels of HPL tend to be highest at that time, but it can be performed earlier if your physician believes that you may develop gestational diabetes—usually because you have a history of endocrine disorders or gestational diabetes in a previous pregnancy. The test is fairly simple: You are given a soda-like beverage to drink and asked to drink it all down within 5 minutes. After 1 hour, blood is drawn, and a reading of blood sugar is taken. Slightly less than 25% of women who undergo this test show signs of having abnormally elevated blood sugar (above 140), but this is a misleading figure—most of these women do not have gestational diabetes, and a 3-hour glucose tolerance test performed later generally sorts out the ones who do have it from the ones who don't. In general, gestational diabetes occurs in only 3% to 5% of all pregnant women.

As mentioned earlier, gestational diabetes is a hormone-driven event related to a hormone secreted by the placenta; therefore, you can expect the diabetes to end when the baby has been delivered and the placenta is no longer present to produce HPL. (If it does not, that probably means you had undiagnosed diabetes before becoming pregnant.) However, if you have gestational diabetes in one pregnancy, your chances of having it again in later pregnancies are quite high, as about

Oral glucose tolerance test

A test to determine how a pregnant woman's body responds to glucose; a gestational diabetes test.

65% of women who have gestational diabetes in one pregnancy have it again in later pregnancies. Also, approximately half of all women who have gestational diabetes will develop type 2 diabetes later in life. This is especially true of women who were obese before becoming pregnant, had very high blood sugar during pregnancy, developed gestational diabetes very early in the pregnancy, or had postpartum glucose tests that were not quite in the range of diabetes, but very close. In any of these cases, talk to your doctor about how to lower your risk for type 2 diabetes through exercise and nutrition after the baby is born.

53. What is preterm labor? Why does it occur?

Preterm labor is when a mother goes into labor prior to the 37th week of pregnancy; this is generally the point at which the baby's lungs and organs have reached their full size and function. If all else has gone well in the pregnancy, going into labor a week or two (or three) before the due date isn't considered a problem unless other complicating circumstances exist (a breech presentation, for example; see Question 55). Giving birth prior to 37 weeks, however, often requires that the baby be cared for in a NICU until he or she is more mature physically, especially concerning lung function.

There are a number of reasons that an obstetrician might consider a patient to be at high risk for preterm labor. The most common of these are listed in Question 22, but they all have a situation in common in which the mother has some sort of health problem that puts a strain on her body's ability to support a pregnancy for the full duration of normal gestation; however, it is not always the case that a patient at risk for preterm labor does go into labor early (only about 30% do), and it is certainly not unusual for a patient with none of the common risk factors to experience preterm labor: About 70% of all preterm labors occur in women with no known risk factors.

54. What triggers preterm labor? Can preterm labor be stopped?

Any number of circumstances can trigger preterm labor, even in an otherwise healthy woman, but two stand out: stress and dehydration. Stress is thought to trigger preterm labor by inducing the body to release hormones, specifically corticotrophin-releasing hormone (CRH), which can encourage uterine contractions; however, stress is difficult to quantify, and of course, all people respond differently to stressful situations. CRH is also produced by the placenta, so it is thought that this hormone may play a role in determining when the onset of labor occurs; if CRH levels are boosted beyond a certain point because of stress, the body may respond by going into labor. Similarly, dehydration (another fairly common cause of premature labor) triggers an inadvertent hormonal response in the uterus. When a pregnant woman becomes dehydrated, her uterine contractions increase, although we don't really know why.

Most preterm contractions aren't labor.

Contractions in and of themselves don't necessarily signal preterm labor, and indeed, most preterm contractions *aren't* labor. Preterm contractions can sometimes be stopped if the mother is able to recognize the signs relatively quickly and take action (see Question 59). If you are showing signs of possible preterm labor, your doctor will tell you to drink a glass of water (to combat dehydration) and to lie down and rest (to reduce stress, as well as to limit the pull of gravity on the fetus). Either of these actions, taken relatively quickly after symptoms begin, can potentially halt contractions; however, should contractions progress to full preterm labor, medications, primarily corticosteroids, to temporarily halt contractions may be used (see Question 76), allowing the doctors to prepare for the baby's premature birth. Unfortunately, no way is currently available to halt preterm labor completely after it has begun.

Even if you and your doctor successfully stop an episode of preterm contractions, you will need to be alert for another episode. Your doctor will probably advise you to pay close attention to your hydration and rest and may perform a **fetal fibronectin test** to help determine whether you're truly at high risk of true labor (the test looks for increased presence of the "glue" that attaches the fetal sac to the uterus; if it's there in high amounts, it's a sign that labor may be imminent). If signs point to a high likelihood of impending preterm labor, your doctor may recommend bed rest or, at the very least, that you stop working and decrease your overall activity levels so that you will not go into labor again until you are closer to your due date, particularly if the premature contractions occurred before the 37th week. Corticosteroid medications may be prescribed to speed up the maturing process of your baby's lungs, as described in Question 82.

Fetal fibronectin test

A blood test that measures levels of the "glue" holding the fetus in the uterus to determine whether labor may be imminent.

55. What complications might occur during labor? Is there any way to predict or prevent them?

You've gotten all the way through your pregnancy (with or without complications). Your due date is at hand, and you're finally in labor. The birth of your long-awaited baby is imminent . . . and something goes wrong. Your cervix won't dilate. Your contractions falter midway through, or maybe your baby is coming toes first instead of head first—many, many situations can occur at the last minute. Take heart and don't panic: labor complications rarely result in serious danger to either mother or baby, and even when such situations arise, they usually can be resolved.

There are two types of labor complications: either the mother's body responds improperly to labor or some factor related to the baby or placenta interferes with the safe passage of the baby through the birth canal.

MATERNAL COMPLICATIONS

In an otherwise healthy mother, complicated labor most often occurs in first-time mothers and older mothers. One very common situation occurs when contractions and cervical ripening (dilation and effacement) do not occur in tandem: Either the contractions start but the cervix does not dilate, or the cervix is fully dilated and effaced but no contractions are occurring. The latter can be particularly problematic if the amniotic sac ruptures without the contractions starting within 24 hours, as this creates a risk of **cord prolapse** (the umbilical cord slips out of the uterus in advance of the baby, potentially interfering with the baby's blood supply).

Cord prolapse

A situation in which the umbilical cord slips out of the uterus in advance of the baby, potentially interfering with the baby's blood supply

In such cases, the first step is to try to jump start whichever process is stalled. For a cervix that isn't "ripe"—dilated (opened) and effaced (softened and shortened)—synthetic prostaglandins such as dinoprostone or misoprostol are administered to encourage the cervix to ripen. Another medication, pitocin (a synthetic form of the labor-inducing hormone oxytocin), is sometimes given for cervical ripening, but it is used more for mothers whose labor hasn't gotten fully under way because it also causes contractions to increase in frequency and force.

If the cervix is ripe and the baby's head is fully engaged in the pelvis but no contractions have begun—particularly if the due date has passed by a week or more—the obstetrician may induce labor. The simplest way to do this is to break the amniotic sac, which usually triggers the start of contractions; however, if the sac breaks on its own without contractions starting—or if breaking the sac artificially doesn't start them within 24 hours—other methods may be used. Use of a warm whirlpool bath often works, or intravenous pitocin or vaginal misoprostol may be given to encourage uterine contractions. Monitoring of contractions is crucial with these medications, as overly strong contractions are a problem for the baby.

Women who have other health problems, particularly problems related to high blood pressure, are also more likely to have complications. Most of the time, vaginal birth can still take place in a mother with mild to moderate health issues (that is, a chronic illness such as asthma, diabetes, or hypertension, assuming that it is reasonably well controlled), but some assistance may be needed in the form of supplemental oxygen or other supportive measures. Her labor will be monitored carefully to make sure that it is not overtaxing her strength or stressing the fetus; however, health problems in the mother can limit her ability to withstand the stresses of labor. If the labor is prolonged and difficult and no progress is made despite using medications, the obstetrician will recommend a cesarean section. If there are foreseeable problems with vaginal delivery (a big baby in a mother with a narrow pelvis, for instance), the obstetrician may recommend a cesarean even before labor begins (see Question 83). Labor generally averages about 20 hours for first-time mothers, although it's often quicker in later pregnancies.

Elizabeth's comment:

In my first pregnancy, I'd had complications throughout, so when I finally went into labor, it was a relief . . . finally done with boring bed rest! Then it became clear that the contractions were not dilating the cervix. Even rupturing the membranes didn't help much. I went home and had my acupuncturist give me treatments to slow down the contractions in the hope that if we "started over" we could coax the cervix to dilate. Five hours later, I went back to the hospital to find that I'd dilated only 2 centimeters. It was enough to admit me, but not enough to get the show on the road. Frustrating!

This went on for a very long time—it was 17 long hours of walking, whirlpool baths, sitting on a birthing ball, and every other known strategy. I was tired and becoming scared that I would wind up in surgery having a c-section, something I really wanted to avoid. Although I'd held off on having an epidural (out of concern that it would slow down my labor, ironically enough), there was little choice at this point: I couldn't tolerate the pain any longer and needed to rest. The baby wasn't in any distress according to the fetal monitors, so the big concern was whether I'd have the strength to push when the time came. My doctor suggested we use a shot of pitocin to help with dilation and an antibiotic because I'd started running a fever—all of that work had kicked a low-grade sinus infection into high gear. The epidural all but stopped the contractions, but it brought enough relief to allow me to sleep a few hours. When I woke, the pitocin had done its thing: We were ready to go, and I was rested enough to do my part. One hour later, my son was born—a full 33 hours after I'd first started having regular contractions.

So how do you get through a complicated, marathon labor? Everyone is different, of course, but I think the greatest obstacle many women have in making decisions about how to proceed when complications occur is fear of the unknown or fear of the worst-case scenario. We're all scared that things will go badly, and it's hard to remember that most of the time, childbirth goes well—we're built for it, after all!—but if you can eliminate fear, half your work is done.

FETAL COMPLICATIONS

Some fetal complications are known before labor, and often a cesarean section is scheduled to eliminate the risks—some of them quite serious (see Question 83). Other complications arise just before or during labor. The baby's position in the birth canal, for example, can complicate labor. **Breech birth**, in which the baby enters the birth canal with the feet, knees, or buttocks leading the way and the rest of the baby following, is the most serious form of this type of complication. Although possible when the baby is not positioned head-first, vaginal delivery is generally more difficult, and there is an increased risk of cord prolapse and other harmful complications. For these reasons, most medical and obstetrical organizations

Breech birth

Birth in which the baby is not head down in the birth canal but is positioned feet or buttocks first.

recommend a cesarean section. A baby who is "sunny-side up" instead of in the usual face-down position causes **back labor**. Back labor is not particularly dangerous, but it can be excruciatingly painful and may tire the mother faster; if she is unable to push because of fatigue, the attending doctor or nurse/midwife may need to assist delivery using a vacuum extractor or forceps (although this is fairly uncommon).

Back labor

Labor in which the baby is positioned facing up rather than down.

PART SIX

Symptoms to Watch

How can I tell the difference between normal symptoms and those that need special attention?

What are common symptoms of high blood pressure?

What are the symptoms of preterm labor? How can I distinguish preterm labor from Braxton-Hicks contractions?

More . . .

56. How can I tell the difference between normal symptoms and those that need special attention?

It is difficult in a high-risk pregnancy to know when to pay attention to a symptom. Particularly if this is your first pregnancy, you don't know what's "normal"—and as any pregnancy book will tell you, what's "normal" for one pregnancy isn't the "normal" for another. Even successive pregnancies in the same woman can differ greatly!

Here are a few general rules. First, if the symptoms make you feel debilitated—weak, exhausted, unable to function even to a minimum level, disoriented—you should notify your doctor, even if they seem to be "classic" pregnancy-related symptoms. For example, consider nausea and vomiting. Many, if not most, women experience morning sickness beginning at 8 weeks, and often, the nausea can be severe—occurring both day and night, and resulting in repeated bouts of vomiting through the day; this is considered normal. However, there are many abnormal situations that can mimic standard pregnancy-related nausea and vomiting. For example, some women's nausea is so severe that the pregnancy is adversely affected—a condition called **hyperemesis gravidarum**. The mother begins to lose weight, will likely become dehydrated, and may vomit bile or blood if untreated. This is risky for both mother and fetus and should be addressed quickly. Likewise, if the ordinary first-trimester nausea has faded (as expected) but suddenly returns and/or becomes severe, this is not simply standard morning sickness—something else may be going on. You should alert your doctor. Nausea that begins after the first trimester is also unusual and should prompt a call to your obstetrician.

Hyperemesis gravidarum

Excessive vomiting during pregnancy.

Second, these symptoms may be warning signs that should not wait until your next regularly scheduled checkup:

- A severe, sudden headache
- Vomiting large amounts of mucus, bile, or blood

- Vomiting small amounts food/drink, particularly if you are never able keep anything down
- Rapid weight loss (2+ pounds per week)
- Blood flowing from the vagina (more than "spotting")
- Constipation (if severe)
- Fainting
- Rapid heart rate or palpitations
- Confusion
- Abdominal pain
- Fever

If any of these symptoms occur suddenly—over the course of one to a few days—it is important to report them to your doctor quickly.

Elizabeth's comment:

If any situation is questionable to you, bring it up with your doctor, even if only to get reassurance that all is well. My thyroid problem in my second pregnancy came to light almost accidentally, when Dr. Pinette ended a checkup with the question, "Is there anything else that concerns you?" I was about to say "no," when I suddenly remembered I'd been having occasional heart palpitations. I hadn't really gotten overly excited about them because I knew that the heart works harder during pregnancy, but I brought them up anyway, feeling a little like a hypochondriac. The question inspired him to have my thyroid hormone tested. It was low—not low enough to be a major concern, but still something that needed to be addressed.

57. What are common symptoms of high blood pressure?

Mild hypertension may not have any obvious symptoms, which is why you need to have regular checkups and urinalysis. Symptoms of moderate to severe hypertension include a gradual development of recurring headaches; sudden or severe swelling in the feet, calves, or especially the face and hands; sudden weight gain; blurred vision; malaise or fatigue;

nausea/vomiting; a "band" of pain around the upper abdomen, or alternately a sharp pain in the upper right quadrant of the abdomen (where the liver is located); and sweating in the palms or tingling in the fingers and toes. You may have some or all of these symptoms, but any one of them should prompt a call to your doctor.

Elizabeth's comment:

In my first pregnancy, I had PIH, and very quickly I learned how to tell my when blood pressure was up: My ankles would swell, and I'd feel feverish. My face would become flushed as if I'd been running a race. The minute that happened, I drank water, put my feet up, or lay down, and it would gradually ease. As time passed, however, this occurred more frequently as my regular checkups showed worsening blood pressure. There was a benefit from the experience: When it happened again early in my second pregnancy, I knew what it was—and I knew that I needed to get checked out FAST.

58. What should I do if I experience symptoms of high blood pressure?

First, call your doctor, and discuss the symptoms with him or her; he or she will likely want to see you right away. If you must wait for a few hours or days, however, there are some things you can do to keep your blood pressure stable. First, if necessary, ask your boss if you can take sick time for a couple of days until you can get in to see your doctor. Next, raise your feet higher than your heart, either by putting them up on a footstool or by lying down. If you lie down, lie on your left side—this maximizes blood flow to the fetus as well as reducing the strain on your own heart. Finally, remember to drink 48 to 64 ounces of water each day. Staying well hydrated is key!

59. What are the symptoms of preterm labor? How can I distinguish preterm labor from Braxton-Hicks contractions?

Unfortunately, at first, preterm labor and Braxton-Hicks contractions feel pretty much the same. If you experience ANY contractions, first, have a glass of water, as dehydration can sometimes trigger premature labor, and second, keep track of how often the contractions come, how long they last, and whether there's any particular pattern to them (that is, whether they come only if you stand up or lie down). If they go away after a short while or are irregular, they probably are Braxton-Hicks contractions. Keep monitoring them, but don't let yourself get too upset—they are a normal and necessary part of pregnancy. The uterus needs to exercise and "practice" for the big day. Because the contractions lack rhythm or regularity, they do not cause the cervix to open, as contractions do in true labor. If, on the other hand, they increase in frequency or severity or don't go away if you change position or drink water, then call your doctor. It's better to call unnecessarily than to ignore a real need because you fear being mistaken. If at any point you have bleeding or fluid coming from your vagina, call your doctor *immediately*.

These other signs of preterm labor should inspire a call to your doctor:

- Regular cramping pains, more than five in 1 hour
- Swelling or puffiness of the face or hands
- Pain during urination
- Sharp or prolonged stomach pain
- Vomiting
- A low, dull backache
- Intense pelvic pressure
- Ruptured membranes

60. Should I mention shortness of breath to my doctor?

You are "breathing for two" now; thus, some breathlessness is to be expected in pregnancy, particularly late in pregnancy when your lungs are compressed by the expanding uterus. Any symptom that causes discomfort, however, should be mentioned to your doctor. He or she will question you about related symptoms and perform pulmonary function tests if warranted. If you already have a lung disorder or are suffering a respiratory infection, it is especially important that you let your doctor know that you are experiencing breathlessness. As noted in Question 32, low oxygen levels during pregnancy affect the baby sooner and more severely than the mother, so it's important to address them quickly.

Elizabeth's comment:

It is your God-given right as a pregnant woman to complain about anything and everything to your doctor. So do it! Unless you tell the doctor how you feel, there's no way he or she can get a good picture of what's going on, and in high-risk pregnancy, the docs need to know even the problems you might consider too minor to mention.

61. How much movement is normal for my baby? How can I tell if the baby is "in distress," and when should I call my doctor about the baby's movements?

All babies have different "normal" activity levels. There really is no set standard—you will learn what your baby's usual patterns are as your pregnancy proceeds (it will be easier to feel them after about week 22). After feeling movement, make note of when and how often they occur; keeping a little notebook or a file on a computer can be helpful. You may soon find that your baby has particular times of the day (or night, unfortunately for your ability to rest) that he or she is highly active and other times when you feel nothing at all—probably because the baby is asleep. After a few weeks of monitoring, you should have a pretty good idea of when to expect the baby to be awake and moving.

Your baby should continue to be active on a regular basis for the duration of the second and third trimesters. In the later part of the third trimester, the kicks may be less frequent or less intense, but this isn't necessarily a sign of distress—more likely, this means that the baby's cramped quarters are limiting his or her ability to move. Also, the baby may be moving most when you aren't awake. Squirming, pushing, twitching, and hiccuping may also occur, but as long as you are feeling regular motion, there is no need to be concerned.

Immediately alert your doctor if you feel *no* movement during a time in which you normally would expect to feel it, particularly if you've felt nothing despite attentively waiting for activity or if the baby starts making sudden, frantic, sustained kicks. At the risk of sounding alarmist, let us repeat this: If your baby has moved regularly until now but then suddenly begins moving less or not at all, *call your doctor!* Prompt action when you suspect distress could save your baby's life.

62. How do I know whether the swelling in my hands and ankles is a sign of a complication?

Swelling or **edema** in the legs and feet is common and should be a matter of concern only under the following circumstances:

Edema

Swelling caused by collection of fluid under the skin.

- Swelling occurs suddenly and progresses rapidly; that is, if an hour ago your ankles were their normal size and now they're double in circumference, call your doctor.
- Swelling is excessive and does not decrease when you put your feet up or rest for several hours. Tight shoes at the end of a long day on your feet are nothing to worry

about, but if you get up in the morning and they're still tight, there's probably something wrong.

- Swelling is accompanied by other symptoms such as severe headache, blurred vision, abdominal pain, or a feeling of being overheated that isn't related to the temperature of the room.
- Swelling occurs not only in the feet and legs, but also in the face and hands.

If you experience any of these symptoms, report them to your doctor immediately.

63. Why does my doctor ask about my vision?

Significant vision changes can be a fairly sensitive indicator of an arising problem, usually hypertension or gestational diabetes. Do not feel alarmed if you're having a little trouble seeing far away or close up or if your eyes are dry or itchy. These are fairly common symptoms and are related to the excess fluid in your body, which can slightly alter the shape of your eyes and thicken your corneas. Lubricating drops can help dry eyes, and switching from contact lenses to glasses for the duration of your pregnancy can ease irritation related to changes in the shape and thickness of the cornea. The swelling we discussed in the previous question also can greatly affect your eyes, as can the constriction of blood vessels that occurs in hypertension, so if you notice a *sudden* significant blurring of your vision, if you see spots, flashes, or "waviness," or if you're experiencing tunnel vision (where your peripheral vision disappears), call your doctor, particularly if the change occurs suddenly. Any of these symptoms may be a result of swelling and vasospasm that signal rising blood pressure, which could be related to preeclampsia or diabetes.

64. Why should I tell my doctor if my skin itches?

You might develop itchy skin during pregnancy for several reasons. Your skin may be dry and simply need moisturizer (especially during cold, dry, winter weather); however, a few conditions are specific to pregnant women that cause itchiness—often severe, and sometimes accompanied by a rash. Most of these are not truly harmful to you or your baby, although they might drive you a little nuts, but one condition, **intrahepatic cholestasis of pregnancy (ICP)**, characterized by itchy skin, can be very dangerous to pregnant women. It is extremely uncommon, affecting less than 1% of all pregnant women in the United States (roughly 7 out of 1,000).

Intrahepatic cholestasis of pregnancy is a liver problem in which bile doesn't flow normally in the liver's small ducts, causing it to accumulate in the skin and leading to itching. It generally develops during the third trimester, although it occasionally starts as early as 20 weeks. ICP most often starts on the palms of the hands and soles of the feet. Other symptoms include fatigue, a loss of appetite, and dark urine; a rash is rarely present. In some cases, pregnant women with this condition develop **jaundice** (a yellowing of the skin). Most of the time, these symptoms resolve when the baby is delivered; nevertheless, a woman diagnosed with ICP has a strong chance of having ICP again in later pregnancies. ICP is not generally considered dangerous to the mother's life or long-term health.

ICP is quite dangerous to the baby's health, however. Because your baby has only a limited ability to remove bile acids from the blood—for the most part, it relies on your liver to perform this function—the potential effects of ICP on the baby are extremely serious, even deadly. When ICP occurs before 36 weeks, treatment involves using anti-itch medications to address the symptoms along with a medication called ursodeoxycholic acid (Actigall), which helps correct liver function abnormalities. Some studies suggest that this drug also may help prevent stillbirth (see Question 97); however, your doctor will likely want to monitor the baby closely, possibly inducing delivery at 36 weeks if the baby shows signs of distress.

Intrahepatic cholestasis of pregnancy (ICP)

A liver disorder in which bile doesn't flow properly through ducts in the liver, causing itchy skin and potentially life-threatening complications.

Jaundice

Yellowing of the skin.

Early delivery in this instance is usually less dangerous to the baby's health than ICP. In extreme cases, it may be necessary to promote faster lung development and deliver the baby early, rather than risk the possibility of stillbirth.

A much more common cause of skin itchiness is a condition called **pruritic urticarial papules and plaques of pregnancy (PUPPP)**—a tongue-twister of a term that simply means you have an itchy rash consisting of hives and other skin eruptions. Like ICP, PUPPP generally begins in the second or third trimester, but a PUPPP rash usually starts on the abdomen (particularly on stretch marks) and spreads to the torso, arms, and legs; only rarely is it present on the palms of the hands or soles of the feet, which distinguishes it from ICP. It won't harm either you or your baby, although severe PUPPP can seem nearly unbearable. You probably won't be able to sleep well and may become irritable simply because the itching is so intense. The causes of PUPPP are unknown, and the usual cure is delivering the baby (although a few women continue to have PUPPP for a short time after the baby is born). A few tried-and-true remedies will alleviate PUPPP completely; some work and others don't—still others work for a short time but for various reasons either lose effectiveness or must be discontinued. The Appendix includes a list of Web sites and resources for dealing with PUPPP.

Even if you think it's PUPPP, tell your doctor about it anyway—he or she will most likely want to do a blood test to check for the presence of high levels of bile acids and certain liver enzymes. This is especially important if you have an immediate relative—your mother, aunt, or sister—who has ever had ICP or if you or your ancestors are from Chile, Bolivia, Scandinavia, and China, where ICP is somewhat more common. About half of the women who develop ICP have a family history of related liver disorders. If any of these factors apply to you, get your itchiness checked out. Even if you're not from one of the higher risk groups, for your own peace of mind, you should rule out ICP altogether.

Pruritic urticarial papules and plaques of pregnancy (PUPPP)

An itchy rash that occurs in pregnancy for unknown reasons.

Elizabeth's comment:

I had PUPPP in both my pregnancies, and in both cases, my doctor ordered a blood test to check for bile acids and liver enzymes. The first time I was completely ignorant about either ICP or PUPPP and had no idea why my doctor was so concerned about what I thought was a case of hives—something I get on occasion even when not pregnant. It was a bit unnerving to find out that my "itchies" could be yet another complication in an already complicated pregnancy! During the second pregnancy, I understood about ICP and went into my checkup armed with the knowledge that (1) my doctor would probably order a blood test to check for bile acids and (2) the blood test would probably turn up negative, as I had all the classic signs of PUPPP and none of the symptoms, aside from the itching, of ICP. My doctor—not the same one as before, but still fairly experienced in such things—didn't disappoint me: the first words out of his mouth after looking at my rash were, "We're going to do a blood test, just to be sure," which is about what I'd expected. Also as expected, the test was negative. It was just another case of PUPPP, which is not a day at the beach by any means, but it's a lot easier to deal with going crazy from the itching when you know your baby isn't in danger.

65. Should I be concerned about vaginal discharge or blood spotting?

Most of the time, an increase in vaginal discharge during pregnancy is nothing to worry about. A small amount of milky discharge called **leukorrhea** is common in nonpregnant women, and during pregnancy, this continues, although it may occur in greater amounts. It is normal and is nothing to worry about. Use panty liners or a pad to absorb it, but do not use tampons—a tampon can introduce bacteria into the cervix and cause an infection.

Leukorrhea

Milky vaginal discharge.

If the discharge is yellow, green, or gray, smells foul, or is frothy, you may have a yeast infection. Even if you've treated yeast infections yourself before, don't just reach for a tube of Monistat. Call your doctor first.

Brownish or reddish "spotting" (due to the presence of small amounts of blood) may be a symptom of infection, but because there are more serious situations that could lead to spotting, call your doctor promptly if it occurs before 37 weeks, as it could be related to premature labor. A thin, watery discharge that is tinged with blood may signal rupture of the membranes. Also call your physician in this situation. A thick clot of blood-tinged mucus may be released when the cervix begins to dilate; some pregnancy books refer to this as the "cervical plug," but in reality, it is just mucous ooze and doesn't really mean very much. It is not dangerous, nor does it necessarily mean labor is imminent, although you might want to get your bags packed for the trip to the hospital. Let your doctor know about it, but don't expect that he or she will want to see you. On the other hand, outright vaginal bleeding—even small amounts of bright red blood—is not normal under any circumstances and is a signal that you need to be evaluated immediately. Call your doctor; if he or she is not immediately available, you will likely be advised to go to the nearest hospital's emergency department.

66. As a migraine sufferer, how can I tell the difference between a standard migraine and a headache that could indicate a pregnancy-related complication?

Migraines generally include characteristic effects that don't occur with headaches related to, for example, an episode of very high blood pressure in a pregnant woman. Migraine often includes visual effects such as spots, tunnel vision, or "aura" and may also experience "pins and needles" sensations, which is not normally the case with nonmigraine headaches. Nausea, vomiting, and sensitivity to light and noise are also hallmarks of migraine headaches. Unlike other types of headache, migraines typically cause pain on only one side of the head.

Table 7   Headaches in Pregnancy

Causes
- Hormones
- Lack of sleep
- Dehydration
- Caffeine/nicotine withdrawal
- Low blood sugar
- Tension/stress
- Poor posture
- Sinusitis/congestion
- Migraine
- Head injury
- Preeclampsia/hypertension

Pain Relief Strategies
- Use acetaminophen for pain relief as advised by your doctor. Ibuprofen may be used prior to the third trimester, but consult your doctor before using it, as some patients should avoid NSAIDs. *Do not use aspirin.* Prescription medications for migraine should be discussed with your doctor prior to using.
- Drink plenty of fluids and eat a small, nutritionally balanced meal to combat dehydration/low blood sugar.
- Treat headaches related to sinus/congestion with a warm compress to the eyes and nose. Use decongestants to alleviate congestion as advised by your doctor, or use a saline nasal spray to flush out mucus. Menthol rubs on the forehead above your nose (i.e., above the sinuses) and below each nostril may help open congested nasal passages.
- Treat tension headaches with a cold ice pack at the base of the neck, and have your partner massage your shoulders and neck.
- Treat migraine with a cold compress on your head, rest, and biofeedback while removing or avoiding any trigger factors.
- For tension or sinus headaches, take a warm shower or bath; for migraine, take a cold shower.
- Rest in a dark room, meditate, or practice yoga or other relaxation techniques.
- Acupuncture.

Call Your Doctor If:
- Your headache is accompanied by any of the following: fever, stiff neck, swelling of face/hands, sudden weight gain, abdominal pain, slurred speech, numbness, nausea/vomiting, or blurred/disturbed vision.
- Your headache persists for more than a few hours, returns frequently, or won't go away.
- You develop a headache for the first time in the second or third trimester of your pregnancy and you have already been diagnosed with a hypertensive disorder.
- You have a sudden, explosive headache, one that feels unlike any other you've ever had, or one that wakes you from sleep.
- You have a severe headache after hitting your head.
- You experience vision changes.

Symptoms to Watch

Migraines tend to be triggered by specific events, hormones, or foods, and if you do not have experience with migraines, you may be unaware of what triggers your migraines. Indeed, women who never previously suffered from migraines may first experience it during pregnancy because of hormonal shifts. The pain of migraine is described as "throbbing" and characteristically starts off dull but escalates to pain severe enough to affect speech and mental functioning that lasts from about 4 to 6 hours (although some unfortunate sufferers have migraines lasting as long as 72 hours). The good news? True migraines typically improve during pregnancy.

A headache that is part of a pregnancy-related complication differs from a migraine. First, it is more persistent than a migraine, lasting longer and recurring more often than is normal for migraines. Second, it is often more abrupt; when a migraine will develop from a dull throb to extreme pain, the headaches that occur with complications of pregnancy tend to be sharp and rapid in onset. Migraines are usually relieved with medications such as acetaminophen, Imitrex, or Fioricet or by nonmedicinal techniques (see Table 7), but a nonmigraine headache related to pregnancy complications generally does not respond as well to pain relief, either medicinal or nonmedicinal. You can expect to feel relief from medications within 20 to 30 minutes if the headache is truly a migraine; if you don't, call your doctor. Headaches accompanied by swelling of the hands and face, blurred vision, or abdominal pain (particularly in the upper right quadrant, where your liver is located) should be promptly reported to your doctor.

PART SEVEN

Prevention and Treatment of Complications

Should I avoid certain foods or medications?

Are injections to prevent preterm labor effective?

Why do I need to have so many ultrasound exams?

What is meant by bed rest? What can I do on bed rest?

More . . .

67. Why did my doctor prescribe a prenatal vitamin?

Prenatal vitamin

A vitamin formulated to suit the needs of pregnant women.

Most physicians will prescribe a **prenatal vitamin** soon after you are confirmed pregnant. Some will even prescribe it before pregnancy if they know you're trying to become pregnant. Prenatal vitamins tend to be loaded with vitamins and minerals that many women don't get enough of—B-complex vitamins such as folate and folic acid in particular (see Question 68), as well as iron. Thus, women are encouraged to support their overall health by getting enough of these vitamins via supplements. A prescription supplement is used because they have higher levels of the particular vitamins and minerals that pregnant women need. The risk of complications such as iron-deficiency anemia (see Question 39) can be greatly reduced by using these supplements, as can certain birth defects such as spina bifida and other neural tube defects (see Question 33). Unfortunately, prescription prenatal vitamins can sometimes upset your stomach—most of the time, if you take it just before bedtime, you won't be bothered by nausea or stomach upset. If this doesn't work, let your doctor know—he or she can prescribe a different formulation of prenatal vitamins. It's important to get sufficient levels of these vitamins and minerals each day, so don't give up on the vitamins if they make you feel sick; work with your doctor to find a vitamin supplement that you can manage.

68. Should I take extra folic acid?

Folic acid and its alternate form, folate, also called vitamin B9, are found in leafy green vegetables, fruits, beans, and nuts—many of the foods we're often told we should eat more often than we routinely do. According to the U.S. Centers for Disease Control, most women, pregnant or not, get insufficient folic acid in their diets and should supplement their intake, either through vitamin supplements or by eating fortified breads or cereals.

Folic acid and folate help form healthy new cells; therefore, increased amounts would be helpful to a pregnant woman and her fetus. Most prenatal vitamins (and indeed, most standard over-the-counter multivitamins formulated specifically for women) include about 400 micrograms of folic acid, which is generally sufficient even in pregnancy. If you take such a supplement daily—not just occasionally—there is no reason for additional supplements.

Most obstetricians would recommend increasing the dose above the 400-microgram level only when a woman has already had a pregnancy in which a neural tube defect, such as spina bifida or anencephaly, caused a miscarriage or stillbirth. Such birth defects of the brain and spine are related to low levels of folic acid in the mother; unfortunately, these complications most often occur in the first few weeks of pregnancy. After that time, it may already be too late to prevent those birth defects. Thus, the first step for preventing a recurrence is verifying that the mother has ample stores of folic acid in her system—most easily accomplished by using high-dose supplements. Studies suggest that 3,000 to 5,000 micrograms of folic acid daily reduce the risk of cleft palate, neural tube defects, and certain heart defects; however, excess amounts of folic acid—more than 1,000 micrograms daily—serve no purpose if you're not at risk.

69. Should I avoid certain foods or medications?

The vast majority of foods and medications are safe when you are pregnant, but a few should be limited or skipped entirely.

1. *Raw or cold meat.* Uncooked seafood, undercooked ("rare") beef or poultry, smoked fish or meat, or sliced deli meats can be contaminated with bacterial pathogens such as *Listeria, Toxoplasmosis, E. coli, Salmonella,*

and other disease-causing organisms. Most obstetricians recommend that pregnant women avoid them entirely (see Question 29).

2. *Raw eggs.* Homemade mayonnaise or dressings, custards, and cookie dough containing raw eggs are off the menu—raw, unpasteurized eggs may be contaminated with *Salmonella.* Any such products sold in packaged foods (cookie dough ice cream, for example) are generally safe because eggs used commercially have been pasteurized.

3. *Soft cheeses and unpasteurized milk products.* Milk that has not been pasteurized may be contaminated with *Listeria,* which causes miscarriage. Soft cheeses may likewise be contaminated unless the packaging states that they have been made from pasteurized milk.

4. *Fish.* Concerns about fish stem from the fact that many fish and shellfish contain trace amounts of mercury, a toxin that is particularly dangerous for the developing nervous system of a fetus; however, studies of women who normally eat high quantities of fish have shown no signs that these trace amounts pose a significant threat to the fetus. Given that eating fish has tremendous health benefits, eating one meal of fish per week is likely a healthy choice, but be careful about what you choose. Ocean fish such as albacore tuna, mackerel, and swordfish are particularly high in mercury, but shellfish and freshwater fish from rivers and ponds may also contain unacceptable amounts depending on local conditions (check with your local EPA branch via the Internet). Go ahead and eat your fish, but limit it to once weekly, and pass on some of the previously discussed ocean fish.

5. *Liver.* This is an excellent source of iron but, unfortunately, contains unsafe amounts of vitamin A, which can cause birth defects. Turn instead to safer sources of iron, such as lean beef, poultry (especially dark meat), and iron-rich vegetables such as beans, tofu, raisins, potatoes, apricots, whole-grain breads, and of course, leafy, dark-green vegetables like spinach.

6. *Unwashed and unpeeled fruits and vegetables.* Ground-grown vegetables, even those organically grown, may absorb organisms such as *Toxoplasmosis* and *E. coli* in the soil or water. Nonorganic fruits and vegetables may also contain chemical pesticides. All fruits and vegetables should be thoroughly washed before eating, and it is best to peel fruits or root vegetables (potatoes, carrots) as well.

7. *Caffeinated beverages.* Recent studies suggest that regular caffeine use may compromise blood flow to the fetus enough to almost double the risk of miscarriage. Because caffeine is both a **diuretic** (that is, causes water loss) and a **vasoconstrictor** (causes narrowing of blood vessels), this finding makes perfect sense. Therefore, cut back to no more than one or two caffeinated beverages a day for the duration of your pregnancy, keeping in mind that coffee and cola are not the only sources—many black and green teas, as well as hot cocoa, all have caffeine (skip the "energy drinks" altogether).

Diuretic
Causing increased urination and fluid loss.

Vasoconstrictor
Causing narrowing of the blood vessels.

There are also some foods that you can include in your diet, but consume them at a different time as your prenatal vitamin because they can interfere with the absorption of important vitamins or minerals such as B vitamins or iron. For example, milk products of any kind contain calcium, which reduces iron absorption—so skip the milkshake and cheese if you have a hamburger. Polyphenols in tea and coffee also hinder iron absorption, and caffeine in either one can increase your blood pressure. Again, separate your tea or coffee intake from your vitamin routine, and switch to decaf while pregnant.

As noted in Question 27, most prescription and nonprescription medications are relatively safe in pregnancy, but you may want to avoid some, depending on your specific circumstances. Talk to your doctor about what is and is not safe. Be aware also that numerous herbs used in herbal teas and homeopathic and alternative medicines affect the uterus and should thus be avoided in pregnancy (Table 8).

Table 8   Herbs to Avoid During Pregnancy*

Herb	Why To Avoid It
American mandrake, black cohosh, blue cohosh, bloodroot, calamus, cascara sagrada, cayenne, dong quai, fennel, feverfew, flax seed, goldenseal, lady's mantle, licorice, make fern, mayapple, mistletoe, passion flower, pennyroyal, periwinkle, poke root, rhubarb, sage, senna, tansy, thuja, thyme, wild cherry, wormwood	These herbs are uterine stimulants that can cause uterine contractions (may start preterm labor or miscarriage).
aloe, buckthorn, docks, meadow saffron	These herbs are muscle stimulants and may also cause uterine contraction (cause miscarriage).
cotton-root bark, yarrow, rue	These herbs promote menstruation (cause miscarriage).
juniper, lavender, marjoram, oregano, rosemary, saw palmetto	These herbs contain alkaloids (essential oils) that can affect hormonal activity or other functions in the mother's body and/or harm the fetus.
ephedra (ma-huang) when used orally	Ephedra can stimulate the heart, increase heart rate, and raise blood pressure.
yohimbe	Relaxes the uterus and may be toxic to the fetus.

*Herbs used in cooking, such as rosemary or fennel, generally represent no danger because they are used in small amounts, but using the same herb in a tea or infusion could be harmful.

70. Are there exercises or activities I should avoid?

As noted in Question 19, exercise is generally good for pregnant women, as long as you keep your pulse rate below 140 and lift no more than 40 pounds of weight; however, some of the changes that occur with pregnancy can make certain types of exercise risky, particularly high-impact exercise. The hormone relaxin, which increases with pregnancy, causes ligaments, tendons, and joints to become loosened in preparation for childbirth. Although beneficial during childbirth, it is hazardous during the weeks and months preceding birth because it increases your susceptibility to sprained ankles, pulled tendons, strained ligaments, and other musculoskeletal injuries—at this time, extra weight in your abdomen throw your balance off-kilter. Even if you have the energy to run or play sports, you really should limit such activities, simply because poor balance and weak joints could result in injury. Substituting a less stressful form of exercise, such as walking or swimming, is highly recommended; contact sports such as basketball or soccer generally should be avoided, particularly after about 16 weeks. Amniotic fluid cushions a fetus only so much, and a good, hard hit to the stomach during a basketball game is dangerous. Activities such as horseback riding, cycling, or gymnastics, all of which can put pressure on the pelvis and lower abdomen, should generally be avoided unless you have been continually engaged in them prior to pregnancy. Even then, they should be scaled back or discontinued as the pregnancy advances. While exercising, listen to your body. If you feel achy, dizzy, fatigued, shaky, or weak, stop what you're doing, drink some water, and rest.

Listen to your body: if you feel dizzy, fatigued, shaky, or weak, stop what you're doing, drink some water, and rest.

Even household chores and work-related tasks can put unacceptable strain on your body when you're pregnant. Sitting for long periods of time in front of the computer at work may not *seem* strenuous, but the pressure on your pelvic nerves, blood vessels, and lower back can aggravate the usual discomforts of pregnancy or even lead to further complications such as blood clots in the legs. Get into a routine of standing up and stretching or walking around periodically. If your job demands greater activity, make sure that your doctor is aware of what your work tasks entail, particularly those that require lifting, stretching, climbing, squatting, or bending. You may need to ask your employer to scale back or eliminate these tasks from your assignment for the duration of your pregnancy—if this is an issue at your workplace, ask your doctor for a detailed description of what activities are and aren't acceptable and why. Most employers will be accommodating, but if they aren't, contact the U.S. Equal Employment Opportunity Commission and file a complaint. Under U.S. law, if you are not able to perform job tasks due to pregnancy, your employer must treat you the same as any other temporarily disabled worker—for example, by providing modified tasks, alternative assignments, disability leave, or leave without pay.

71. Are there medications I can take for cold and flu symptoms that won't harm my baby or exacerbate existing risk factors?

Most obstetricians do not hesitate to suggest common decongestants (even in a woman who is high risk) when a cold or mild flu makes a patient uncomfortable. Most decongestants are fairly safe, and relieving cold symptoms may help the expectant mother get enough rest and eat properly. Nonprescription medications such as pseudoephedrine and phenylephrine HCl can be purchased over the counter. Follow the directions given specifically for pregnant women. Consult your physician if you are on any other medications already, just in case there are side effects or drug interactions that might be a concern.

If you are reluctant to use decongestants, a number of other techniques that have no significant effects on your baby can be used to relieve symptoms. The standard advice to drink lots of fluids when you're sick is vital, particularly if the bug makes you vomit or have diarrhea. Staying hydrated is essential—if you can't keep fluids down for more than a few hours, you should definitely call your doctor, as he or she will want to make sure you do not become seriously dehydrated. Also, during a respiratory infection, the additional fluids help to thin the mucous secretions, making it easier to breathe.

Since there is only so much liquid your overtaxed bladder can hold at this point, you may also wish to use these alternative means of relieving your lungs and sinuses:

- Breathe in steam from a warm shower or a steam inhaler to help open nasal passages and loosen phlegm in the lungs. Do this just before going to bed at night and after waking in the morning. Do *not* use a steam humidifier round the clock or all night, as it can be a breeding ground for bacteria—instead, keep your bedroom and workspace humid using a *cold*-water humidifier instead of a steam-generating humidifier. (We suggest a warm shower, rather than hot, because being overheated while pregnant is not a very good idea, and a warm shower can generate just as much moisture in the air as a hot one.)

- Place a warm, damp washcloth or compress over your eyes and above your nose. The heat will loosen some of the secretions in your sinuses and ease sinus pressure. Also, saline nasal sprays used to "flush" the sinus passages can help relieve stuffiness.

- Use over-the-counter menthol rubs (Vicks VapoRub, for example) or mentholated additives for humidifiers to boost penetration of moisture when you're particularly stuffy. Do *not* use mentholated cough drops—the idea is to inhale the vapors, not ingest them. Menthol rubs are best used at night and rubbed on your upper chest under your clothes; do not put them in your nostrils, as menthol can injure the delicate membranes in your nose.

- If you're feeling well, take a short walk, particularly if it is damp outside. Exercise acts as a bronchodilator (that is, it opens air passages), and walking on a misty or rainy day may help to open your sinuses and lungs. Of course, if you're so miserable you can barely tolerate the walk to the bathroom, this particular strategy isn't for you!

If your symptoms are severe or you feel that you are becoming dehydrated, notify your obstetrician.

72. What is a nonstress test? What can the doctor learn from it?

A nonstress test measures fetal activity in response to conditions in the uterus, particularly contractions, after about week 28 of the pregnancy. It is called a nonstress test because no stressors of any kind aside from the normal conditions in the womb are put on the fetus. These measurements involve the use of monitors that detect the fetal heart rate and uterine contractions, both of which are recorded on a strip of paper (resembling the EKG strips used for heart patients) for a period of 20 to 30 minutes.

Nonstress tests are performed when fetal distress is a possibility. It is a common technique for monitoring fetal health in high-risk pregnancy. During a nonstress test, the doctor or nurse will want to see how the fetus responds to contractions and whether its heartbeat increases and decreases normally during periods of activity versus periods of rest. A sick baby is very similar to a sick adult: He or she prefers to lie around, doing very little. Healthy babies, like healthy adults, move more and have more rapid heart rates when they are active and slower heart rates when resting (but not so slow as to affect blood flow and oxygen levels in the tissues). A healthy baby's heart rate should remain stable during a contraction. A drop in heart rate during Braxton-Hicks contractions or any other deviation from expected normal heart rhythms could be a sign that there is a problem with blood flow through the placenta or umbilical cord and is a principal indicator of fetal distress.

A lack of movement from your baby during a nonstress test isn't necessarily a cause for alarm. As mentioned in Question 61, a fetus has periods of sleep and wakefulness that don't necessarily correspond to its mother's sleep patterns. The nurse supervising the test may use a buzzer or gentle prodding to wake the baby, but that isn't always successful—some babies are sound sleepers! Most "failed" nonstress tests, in our experience, are healthy, lazy babies rather than sick babies. If you can eat a meal or drink some water, juice, or soda shortly before the test, it might help get the baby moving so that the test doesn't simply record a snoozing fetus (and it also prevents you from getting hungry during what might be an hour-long process); however, if you haven't felt any movement in the past day and the test records no significant movement over the course of 30 to 60 minutes, your doctor may order an ultrasound (Question 74).

73. Why does the doctor test my urine at every visit?

This charming ritual of pregnancy is necessary because some of the earliest signs of complications are found in the urine. Glucose in the urine, for example, can signal the onset of gestational diabetes (Questions 50–52) while protein in the urine can indicate impaired kidney function (possibly because of infection or pregnancy-induced hypertension) and, late in pregnancy, may also be associated with preeclampsia (Question 46). Such diagnoses depend, however, on observing glucose and/or protein levels that are *consistent*. That is, if protein shows up in a single urinalysis, it is a red flag that alerts health care providers to the possibility of certain complications, but it doesn't by itself mean that a real problem exists. *Repeated* appearance of abnormal urinalysis results will signal a need for further testing. Thus, urine tests are performed regularly to catch the earliest indicators of potential complications.

74. Why do I need to have so many ultrasound exams?

An ultrasound is the most effective way to monitor the condition of your baby, and in high-risk pregnancy, it ensures that all is well. Using sound waves to create a visual image, the ultrasonographer can "see" into the baby's body and determine whether its organs are functioning properly, measure its growth, determine how much amniotic fluid is present, and check the blood flow through the umbilical cord. A healthy baby practices breathing and explores its world by moving around; observations of such activities form the baby's **biophysical profile**. An ultrasound can also reveal the location and condition of the placenta, as well as verify that the baby is entering the birth canal in the appropriate head-first

Biophysical profile

A collection of measurements taken by ultrasound that assess the baby's health and growth rate.

position. Because conditions in high-risk pregnancy can change, regular fetal surveys are necessary to determine the baby's condition and progress. Your obstetrician is able to watch for early signals of trouble, enabling him or her to take action if complications appear.

75. When should I have my cervix examined?

For the most part, your cervix does not need to be examined routinely unless one or more of the following circumstances applies:

History of incompetent cervix. If your medical history indicates or suggests incompetent cervix (see Question 23), your doctor may check the condition of your cervix, either prior to your pregnancy or during the early weeks of the pregnancy. If the cervix has dilated more than 2.5 cm (1 inch) or if it has **effaced** (shortened) to less than 20 mm (about 3/4 inch) before 35 weeks—and usually much earlier—the diagnosis of incompetent cervix will be suspected. A diagnosis of possible incompetent cervix does not mean that you will automatically lose your baby, nor does it mean that you cannot have other children should you miscarry, but it will mean that you will need to undergo some rather drastic measures to prevent miscarriage or premature birth (see Question 79).

Effaced
Shortened.

Premature contractions, bleeding, or vaginal fluid loss. A cervical exam may be performed if there are concerns about premature rupture of the membranes or the onset of preterm labor signified by premature contractions or fluid or blood loss from the vagina. Checking for cervical dilation can help determine whether preterm labor might be imminent, thus allowing the doctor to take steps to prevent it. Aside from these situations, your doctor will likely examine your cervix at least weekly when you reach full term to check for cervical ripening, one of the early signs of labor.

76. Are injections to prevent preterm labor effective?

At the moment, we would have to answer this question with a rousing "maybe," because it all depends on what you consider to be "effective." Is there a magic potion that will stop labor and allow a baby to stay in place until the pregnancy reaches full term? Definitely not; if there were, we'd have no worries about preterm babies at all. Can we stave off labor for even a short while using medications? Yes—sometimes. As you can see, there are no simple answers here.

Two types of medications are used in women at risk for pre-term labor: **tocolytic medications** that stop contractions that have already begun, and progesterone injections that are used to prevent early labor from occurring. Tocolytic medications include a number of different drugs that can delay true labor on average of a day or two. This delay can be valuable. It allows doctors to treat the mother with corticosteroid medications (see Question 82) and prepare for treatment of the premature infant in a NICU. In some situations, tocolytics cannot be used: if the mother has severe preeclampsia or eclampsia, if the baby is in severe distress, or if the mother's cardiovascular health is unstable. Specific tocolytic medications can't be used when the mother has certain conditions—for example, a medication called nifedipine must be used cautiously in a woman who has liver damage, and another medication called indomethacin can't be used in women with asthma. Therefore, the doctor must have a thorough knowledge of the mother's health history before choosing the medication. If you are at risk of preterm labor and have any significant health issues that could affect which medication can be used safely, discuss the matter with your doctor in advance so that you can let treating physicians know what is and is not safe if you are preterm labor in an emergency room.

Ideally, doctors could prevent preterm labor from starting in the first place. Recent research suggests that in women who

> **Tocolytic medications**
>
> Medications that can temporarily halt premature contractions.

have at least one prior premature delivery with unknown cause, weekly treatment with a synthetic form of progesterone—a hormone naturally produced by the body and produced in high quantities by the placenta—may lower the risk of preterm birth. This treatment was given as weekly intramuscular shots starting at 18 to 20 weeks through the 35th week. Although all of the treated women did not carry full term, in most cases, it extended the pregnancy. The study showed that this treatment reduced the risk of preterm delivery by about 30% to 50%. The type of progesterone used in this research, 17 alpha-hydroxyprogesterone caproate, is not yet approved for preventing premature birth, nor is it readily available in many parts of the country; thus the use of progesterone injections is not always possible.

Good prenatal care and elimination of risk factors in the mother's lifestyle are the best ways to prevent preterm labor.

Currently, good prenatal care and elimination of risk factors in the mother's lifestyle are the best ways to prevent preterm labor. If preterm labor is a significant risk in your pregnancy, the use of progesterone, tocolytics, and other methods of prolonging gestation is something you can discuss with your doctor, understanding that any or all of these methods might or might not work in your particular case.

77. How is gestational diabetes treated?

The goal in treating gestational diabetes is to stabilize the mother's blood sugar levels so that the baby doesn't grow too large, too fast. Managing blood glucose in a mother with gestational diabetes is done by monitoring blood sugar levels at short, regular intervals and responding to high blood sugar with dietary and exercise changes (in mild cases) or insulin injections (in more severe cases).

The first step in treating gestational diabetes is to monitor blood glucose levels. Although some of this is done in your doctor's office through urinalysis, you might also be asked to self-monitor using kits that are available at your pharmacy. Self-monitoring involves pricking your finger to obtain a drop of blood, which you put onto a special strip of paper and feed into a computerized meter. The meter returns a numeric readout of what your blood glucose level is at that time. With help from your doctor, you will know by that readout whether you need to take immediate action to raise or lower your blood glucose. This will help you and your health care team to determine whether any other changes are needed to help control your blood sugar for the long term. Self-monitoring also enables you to learn to recognize how it feels to have high or low blood sugar. After you know the symptoms, addressing blood glucose levels quickly will become much easier.

The second step in treating gestational diabetes is assessing your diet. Getting control of your carbohydrate intake is one of the most important treatments. **Carbohydrates** are simple and complex sugars that contribute directly to blood glucose levels. Although carbohydrates—particularly complex carbohydrates—are necessary in a healthy diet, many people, pregnant or otherwise, who develop diabetes are shocked to discover just how much of their food is composed of carbohydrates. Bread, pasta, potatoes, and especially junk food and sweets are almost entirely composed of carbohydrates, especially simple carbohydrates. Often, reducing blood glucose levels simply means eliminating or reducing some high carbohydrate foods and adding higher protein foods in place of the carbohydrates. If you're unsure about whether your diet is appropriate for gestational diabetes, make a food diary. Write down everything you eat or drink each day for a week, including snacks. When that week is over, divide the foods according to the basic food groups: meat/eggs, dairy, grains, fruits/vegetables, and sweets/snacks (and yes, putting ice cream in the dairy group *is* cheating!) so that you can compare the proportion of each one in your diet. To balance your diet in favor of lower blood glucose, eat mostly foods that are high in protein (meat, eggs, dairy, and beans), with breads (preferably whole grain), vegetables, and fruits composing the remainder. Only a small amount (less than 10%) should

Carbohydrates
Simple and complex sugars and starches in food.

come from the sweets/snacks group. You may need to make some changes; ask your doctor to refer you to a nutritionist, who can help to recommend foods that are lower in sugars (particularly because many packaged foods contain "hidden" sugars) and offer advice on how to restructure your diet. It may seem difficult to make these dietary changes in the midst of pregnancy cravings, but you may be sparing yourself *and* your child some serious complications later on by making the effort now. Furthermore, making the changes now could help you avoid type 2 diabetes later in life.

Exercise is a very important part of the prescription for lowering blood glucose levels for three reasons: First, when you exercise, your muscles burn the glucose in the blood for energy. Second, regular exercise increases the amount of muscle you have, which in turn increases the demand for glucose, keeping blood sugar levels from rising too high. Finally, third and most important, exercise makes insulin more efficient at transporting glucose to the tissues (that is, the insulin in your body can transport more glucose if you exercise than if you don't). If exercise is not something you enjoy, take heart. You need take only a short, brisk walk of 10 to 15 minutes twice each day to receive some of the beneficial effects (if possible, we also highly recommend swimming). After it becomes habit, increase the time to 20 minutes. Then you may find that you have fewer problems with high or low blood sugar—and you might even enjoy it.

If you are unable to exercise because of injury or other health problems or if your blood glucose levels are especially high, you may need to couple dietary changes with insulin injections. Most of the time, your doctor will give these on a regular schedule—you'll not likely need to learn to self-inject insulin the way people with type 1 diabetes do. You will still need to self-monitor your blood glucose levels. Stabilizing your blood glucose should enable you to avoid preterm labor or other complications of gestational diabetes.

78. What is the treatment for PIH and HELLP?

Hypertensive disorders in pregnancy are monitored more than they are treated, as they are "cured" by delivering the baby. Thus, most pregnancies affected by PIH and/or HELLP are managed by regular urine tests, blood tests (looking for liver enzymes, particularly if HELLP is suspected), and ultrasounds to monitor fetal growth and blood flow through the placenta. These tests will give doctors a good indication of when delivery is essential for the well-being of both mother and baby.

The exceptions are those cases in which hypertension develops very early in the pregnancy or is already present beforehand but becomes dramatically worse during the pregnancy—that is, when ordinary hypertension is coupled with PIH, a very serious situation. In such cases, delivery may not be an option because the fetus cannot survive, so treatment to stabilize blood pressure as long as possible, giving the fetus more time to develop, is the goal. The methods used to accomplish this include:

- Incorporating dietary changes in the form of reducing added salt and fats in foods, elimination of caffeine, and maintaining proper hydration
- Getting sufficient rest and keeping feet elevated to reduce the stress on the heart and blood vessels
- Using antihypertensive medications such as methyldopa, labetalol, nifedipine, hydralazine, and less frequently, atenolol and clonidine (other antihypertensive medications, including ACE inhibitors such as enalapril and captopril, diuretics such as furosemide, and the beta-blocker propanolol are not used in pregnancy because of effects they have on the fetus)

These strategies will be used in conjunction with monitoring in an effort to prolong the pregnancy, ideally to week 37, but if that's not possible, then at the very least to the point at which the fetus is capable of surviving in a NICU.

79. I have incompetent cervix. What will my doctor recommend to prevent another miscarriage?

The management of an incompetent cervix will depend on several factors. First, how far along were you in the pregnancy when the diagnosis was made? Second, to what extent had your cervix already dilated at the time of diagnosis? Third, what is your physical condition at the time of diagnosis? (For example, are there any signs of irritation of the cervix or breaking of the amniotic membrane?) Finally, what is the status of the fetus at the time of diagnosis? Is it healthy and growing, in visible distress, or already beyond help?

Cerclage

A procedure in which the cervix is stitched shut to prevent premature opening.

If the diagnosis of incompetent cervix has been made early in the pregnancy (or even before the pregnancy because of previous late miscarriage), one of the principal treatments is a procedure called **cerclage**, in which the cervix is essentially stitched closed until the pregnancy reaches its 37th week. This can be done as a preventative measure at about 12 to 16 weeks in women with known incompetent cervix. In women who have not had a previous diagnosis of incompetent cervix, it can be performed later than this, as long as the cervix has not dilated more than 4 cm, but generally, "the earlier, the better."

Preventative cerclage can be up to 90% effective in preventing loss of pregnancy in women with incompetent cervix. "Rescue" cerclage, used when incompetent cervix is discovered during a pregnancy, works about 50% of the time. However, cervical incompetence is not easy to diagnose accurately, and cerclage performed on women whose history of miscarriage stems from problems other than incompetent cervix is not likely to work as well. If you need a cerclage for your first successful pregnancy, you will not necessarily need it for any subsequent pregnancies; treatment for incompetent cervix sometimes leaves a scar that can alleviate the problem.

Unfortunately, in some circumstances, cerclage can't be used. If your cervix is dilated more than 4 cm or if there is any sort of cervical irritation or inflammation present, cerclage cannot be easily performed. Finally, if your fetus shows signs of distress or if your membranes have ruptured, cerclage probably will not be used, as the management of your pregnancy will need to focus on stabilizing the baby's health as well as preventing premature labor. In cases in which cerclage is not available, the best option for preventing miscarriage or premature delivery is bed rest, as discussed in Question 80.

80. What is meant by bed rest? What can I do on bed rest?

Many doctors treating a woman with high-risk pregnancy will prescribe bed rest. This is a simple prescription that can potentially alleviate certain physiological problems without using drugs or other medical interventions. In certain cases, such as incompetent cervix or high-end multiples, it may be essential to preventing preterm labor or miscarriage.

Unfortunately, there is no hard-and-fast delineation of how bed rest is conducted. Under certain circumstances (usually threatened miscarriage or extreme premature labor), some practitioners recommend **complete bed rest** or **hospitalized bed rest**, which requires that the mother never let her feet touch the floor for any reason, including using the bathroom (a bedpan is used instead). This form of bed rest most often takes place in a hospital or care facility, as it is too demanding for home use. A mother placed on **strict bed rest** may get up to use the bathroom but is otherwise confined to her bed. In both complete and strict bed rest, the mother is often instructed to lie on her left side to optimize blood flow to the fetus. **Modified bed rest** simply requires the mother to stay off her feet as much as possible and keep her body relatively

Complete bed rest

Bed rest in which the mother is forbidden to arise from bed for any reason.

Hospitalized bed rest

Complete bed rest that takes place in a hospital.

Strict bed rest

Confinement to bed except for use of the bathroom.

Modified bed rest

Bed rest in which the mother may get up periodically but should stay in bed most of the time.

horizontal most of the day to minimize cardiovascular stress. Depending on the situation, any of these forms of bed rest may be appropriate to the patient, but much of the time, bed rest is prescribed when it is either unhelpful or inappropriate. To make matters worse, a physician may prescribe "bed rest" without telling the patient what that means!

If you are prescribed bed rest, particularly if it means that you will be laid up for more than a week or two, and especially if you must leave work because of it, do not simply take the prescription (pardon the expression) lying down. Ask your doctor to explain *why* he or she wants you on bed rest. If the answer does not include specific physiological benefits to the fetus or to your overall health (that is, "it will improve fetal blood flow" or "your blood pressure is markedly lower when you're lying down"), argue your case against this strategy. Alternative methods are available for reducing strain on your cardiovascular system and alleviating emotional stress, and these will not entail chaining yourself to your bed, which ultimately might prove more stressful than continuing with your standard activities. If, however, your physician offers good, sound reasons for wanting you off your feet, ask him or her to describe exactly what is and is not permitted under the bed rest regimen. Can you walk to the bathroom? Sit up in bed? Get up for meals or occasional excursions outdoors? Do you need to keep your feet elevated or lie on your left side? Clarifying these details with your physician will save a lot of frustration, particularly if your bed rest is extended.

Elizabeth's comment:

In my first pregnancy, my blood pressure began to rise 10 weeks before my due date. My doctor advised me to take certain steps to lower it—drink water, elevate my feet, limit my salt intake, get more rest, and so forth. She ensured my compliance by hinting that bed rest was in my future if my blood pressure continued to rise. So of course, I took her advice—I was the sole breadwinner in my family and certainly did not want an enforced absence from my job! Unfortunately, all those strategies merely put off the inevitable—week after week, the readings were higher, and finally, 4 weeks before my due date, she insisted that I stop working and go on bed rest. I fought this decision, but she made it clear that I was developing preeclampsia. The stress involved with commuting and working was only making it worse. Moreover, it was obvious from all my nonstress tests that my blood pressure went down considerably when I was lying down. What could I say? Clearly, bed rest was beneficial to me and my baby. Thankfully, it was modified bed rest—I was allowed to get up from time to time. It still made me crazy, but I tried to be thankful for the small things—like being able to check e-mail from time to time.

81. What are the physical effects of prolonged bed rest? Are there benefits to hospitalized bed rest versus bed rest at home?

Extended bed rest may be appropriate under certain circumstances: in cases of incompetent cervix, high-order multiples, or combinations of pregnancy complications that carry a high risk of preterm labor (for example, in a mother carrying twins who has PIH or HELLP syndrome). Unfortunately, there are some drawbacks to extended bed rest, particularly if the mother is required to lie on her left side. Bed sores, cardiovascular deconditioning (that is, a decrease in the efficiency of the heart and lungs because of a lack of exercise), decreased muscle tone, joint pain, blood clots, difficulty sleeping, depression, anxiety, and fatigue are side effects of prolonged bed rest. Most women would agree, however, that the psychological effects of prolonged bed rest are by far the most difficult to cope with. Ultimately, there is no clear evidence to prove that bed rest actually works: Most studies show little or no benefit except in the specific situations listed here.

Hospitalized bed rest has some benefits under extreme circumstances—for example, where the mother's condition requires not only strict bed rest, including the use of a bed pan, and medications, particularly if her partner must work outside the home and/or care for young children. However, disconnection from familiar surroundings and people may add to the emotional strain of the bed rest itself. Hospitalized bed rest may also present a financial burden to families whose insurance may not cover any or all of the rather significant costs involved. Thus, hospitalized bed rest should be used only when necessary.

If your physician recommends hospitalized bed rest, make sure that you understand what his or her rationale is. You do not *have* to agree to it, but listen to his or her reasons. Be aware that the American College of Obstetrics and Gynecology has issued a statement *against* the "routine" use of bed rest as treatment or prevention for preterm labor: Your doctor should prescribe it because he or she truly thinks it's warranted *in your case*, not because it's a "standard" treatment.

82. What are corticosteroid medications used for?

Corticosteroid medications

Medications that can induce production of surfactant in a preterm fetus.

Surfactant

A substance in the lungs that enables lung tissue to move more easily.

Corticosteroid medications such as betamethasone or dexamethasone are used when doctors see evidence that preterm delivery is likely in a pregnancy that is only 24 to 34 weeks along. These medications, injected into the mother, encourage the fetus's lungs to produce **surfactant**, a substance that lubricates the lining of the air sacs in the lungs. Surfactant is produced naturally in full-term babies (35 weeks or older), and using corticosteroids in premature infants to stimulate surfactant production decreases the likelihood of breathing problems after birth as well as brain hemorrhage, intestinal infection, and death. These medications are most effective if the baby is delivered 1 to 7 days after the medication is given to the mother, and repeat doses may provide benefits later.

83. Under what circumstances would my doctor recommend a cesarean?

Cesarean section is normally recommended only when there are good reasons to believe that vaginal birth poses a high risk to the baby, the mother, or both: placenta previa, placental abruption, a prolapsed cord, extreme prematurity, high-order multiples, or babies with known birth defects requiring immediate postnatal intervention (or that hamper the baby's ability to pass through the birth canal). Likewise, if the mother's overall health condition is too fragile to withstand labor or if there is a foreseeable problem with the labor (for instance, gestational diabetes has caused the baby to become very large with a potential for a difficult birth), a cesarean section may be planned in advance. Cesarean birth might also be recommended in mothers with herpes or HIV infection to decrease the possibility that the baby will become infected during the birth process. Most physicians also recommend a cesarean birth when the baby is breech, although others argue that this is not necessary when the doctor is experienced in delivering breech babies (see Question 55).

An **emergency c-section** might be necessary if the mother cannot tolerate the rigors of the birth process—for example, if her blood pressure becomes abnormally high or low or if the labor isn't progressing. When fetal monitors indicate that the baby is experiencing distress during labor, particularly during a prolonged or difficult labor, an emergency c-section is sometimes performed.

Emergency c-section

Cesarean section performed because the mother or baby is in distress or imminent danger.

84. Why is my doctor recommending that we induce labor early? Isn't it unhealthy for the baby to be born prematurely?

It is usually better for the fetus to stay in the uterus the full 40 weeks, but in some circumstances, keeping it in utero can actually be harmful to the baby, the mother, or both. If the mother's health is jeopardized by her pregnancy and if the baby is far enough along to be supported in a NICU, then early delivery might be the safest option for both. This occurs most often in cases in which the mother's blood pressure proves difficult or impossible to control, putting her at imminent danger of liver damage, pulmonary edema (fluid in the lungs), or kidney failure. Any of these is also a serious risk of harm to the fetus, including death.

Premature birth does have a number of drawbacks for the baby, particularly if birth occurs before the 32nd week. As mentioned in Question 82, lung maturity is a particular concern in premature babies, and delivery makes them susceptible to lung infections or breathing problems. "Preemies" are also more likely to have problems with digesting food (breast milk or formula), and they may be too weak to suckle effectively, a problem that is, again, most common in babies born before the 32nd week. They also lack the body fat to maintain a correct body temperature (hence the use of incubators in NICUs). Preemies may be anemic, have low blood pressure, or suffer from jaundice caused by excess **bilirubin** in the bloodstream, a situation that can occur in full-term babies but is particularly common in preemies. Also, the rapid growth of the baby's brain that occurs between 32 and 37 weeks is best done in utero. Finally, premature infants may have vision problems related to abnormal growth of blood vessels in the retina. Thus, induction of labor before the 37th week should not be suggested lightly. It should only be performed if there is no other, safer course of action to preserve your and/or your baby's health.

Bilirubin

A substance produced by the spleen that can be elevated in certain diseases.

85. Under what circumstances would termination of the pregnancy be necessary?

This is the hardest subject to address when dealing with the topic of high-risk pregnancy, because most mothers would do absolutely anything to avoid losing their baby. The moral, religious, ethical, medical, and political debates surrounding the issue of pregnancy termination (abortion) are complex and are not debated here; most people in the medical profession understand their patients' conflicted feelings about the subject because we share them.

It is, however, a sad truth that certain situations occur where there is no hope of survival for the baby; sometimes the pregnancy itself poses an imminent danger to the mother's life, or the mother's health is at a critical stage and cannot support a pregnancy. In such situations, pregnancy termination may be a tragic necessity. Sometimes, terminating a pregnancy that is clearly going to end in loss can put the mother on the road to recovery sooner than waiting for a miscarriage or stillbirth to occur naturally. Finally, a pregnancy termination might be chosen if a fetus has such debilitating birth defects that parents feel they will be unable to care for the child after its birth. The following are examples of situations that would lead to pregnancy termination:

- *Ectopic pregnancy.* This is a circumstance where the embryo implants in the fallopian tube rather than the uterus. The fallopian tube, unlike the uterus, is not "stretchy" and therefore will rupture when the embryo grows too large for it, usually within the first trimester. An ectopic pregnancy is inevitably fatal to the embryo, and a rupture of the fallopian tube could be fatal to the mother. Even if she survives, the fallopian tube may be irreparably damaged. Thus, an ectopic pregnancy must be terminated as soon as it is detected. A ruptured ectopic pregnancy typically causes considerable pain and must be treated with surgical removal of the embryo and repair or tying off of the fallopian tube.

- *Inevitably fatal or severely debilitating birth defects.* Some birth defects are so severe that they are guaranteed to lead to eventual miscarriage, stillbirth, or immediate postnatal death. One such defect is anencephaly, a neural tube defect in which the fetus is missing its skull and most of its brain. As with ectopic pregnancy, there is no hope of survival for an anencephalic fetus. Most anencephalic fetuses are miscarried in the first trimester, but some may persist into the second or even the third trimester, so termination of the pregnancy as soon as the defect is discovered often helps the mother to recover both physically and emotionally. Other birth defects can result in severely debilitated newborns whose quality of life would be considered by many to be poor. When faced with the prospect of caring for a severely handicapped child coupled with the family stresses that often coincide (including job loss, divorce, or difficulty caring for other children), some parents make the very painful decision to stop the pregnancy.

• *Life-threatening medical conditions in the mother.* Very rarely, an acute medical condition in the mother might require termination of the pregnancy in order to save the mother's life by reducing stress on the cardiovascular system. Underlying conditions such as heart disease, renal failure, uncontrollable diabetes or hypertension, or rapidly progressing malignancy (cancer) are generally involved in these decisions.

Several things must be understand about pregnancy termination. First, no physician would recommend this course unless he or she truly believed it to be urgently needed to preserve the mother's health, future fertility, or life. Second, pregnancy termination cannot be undertaken without the mother's consent and understanding of why the procedure is required. Your doctor cannot terminate your pregnancy if you refuse on religious or moral grounds, *even if refusing a termination means that you may die.* Finally, consenting to pregnancy termination is a form of loss and should be grieved as a loss without guilt or blame. As we note in our question on loss (Question 99), *you did nothing that led to this result;* even if termination isn't life-and-death for you personally, you would have likely miscarried anyway. Therefore, the termination simply makes the inevitable occur sooner and with less physical trauma to you. Moreover, you likely can and will conceive again if you desire, and with the help of your obstetrical team, your next pregnancy may have a better outcome.

Elizabeth's comment:

I'll be honest: I did not want to include this question in the book because it's too touchy and complicated for so many people. I consider myself pro-choice, but even I would be in agony over having to make such a decision—so how could I even think about writing about it? During the writing of this book, two things happened: First, I heard a radio call-in show on NPR about genetic testing in which a man (who was clearly distressed) described the decision that he and his wife made to terminate a pregnancy affected by Edwards syndrome, a chromosomal defect with lethal consequences. Some months later, I heard from a friend who had two such misfortunes—her first pregnancy was found to be anencephalic and her second was affected by Edwards syndrome. She, too, decided to terminate both pregnancies so that she could recover more quickly. Hearing both of these stories made me realize that this subject is important to discuss, as anyone reading this book might find herself in the same situation. People in these situations need to know that other people face similar decisions and make the choice to terminate even when it's heartbreaking. Ultimately, the best advice is that it's important to talk to your partner, your doctor, and the people whose opinions you value most. Be honest in weighing your choices—then do what's right for you and your family.

PART EIGHT

Daily Concerns in High-Risk Pregnancy

Are there alternatives to bed rest that would allow me to keep working? Are there resources to help support my family?

I'm so worried about my baby's health that I'm losing sleep, and the stress is making the situation worse. What can I do?

Are support groups or health professionals available for women during a high-risk pregnancy?

More . . .

86. My doctor prescribed bed rest, but I support my family financially. Are there alternatives to bed rest that would allow me to keep working? Are there resources to help support my family?

As mentioned in Question 80, bed rest is often overprescribed, and it can be a significant emotional and financial burden on the family. Make sure that your doctor understands that you are not in a position to follow this prescription unless absolutely necessary. Scaling back or changing your hours, telecommuting, or altering your work responsibilities temporarily might be enough to reduce some of the stresses that have affected your health. If your physician is adamant or if it's obvious that bed rest is necessary (for example, you're carrying high-order multiples or have a history of incompetent cervix), you can do a few things.

First, be certain that you understand the limitations and restrictions of your bed rest. This is essential in determining whether a modified work schedule is possible. If your bed rest includes the ability to sit up and move around and if you have a "desk job" or an administrative position, you might be able to telecommute or work from home, part-time if not full-time. Obviously, if your job requires you to be on site and involves physical strain, this is not possible. Next, determine what workplace benefits are available in case of short-term disability. If you are a member of a union, check with your union representative about short-term disability benefits; if you're not a member, check with those who handle employee health and disability benefits. Short-term disability benefits may apply to pregnancy complications, as this is typically a covered disability. Be aware, however, that short-term disability rarely pays your full income and often includes an exclusionary period; thus, you will need to cut back on your expenses, dip into your savings, or find another means of offsetting the difference between income and expenses. Third, you will also need to ask your doctor to write you a letter confirming the complications. Be sure that your doctor includes the date on which the bed rest must begin, as it affects the date that your disability coverage begins.

If your job doesn't offer short-term disability or if you're un-insured, ask your doctor to refer you to a hospital caseworker, who will help you find various government agencies that might have helpful programs. Most hospitals have an experienced, knowledgeable staff that can help with a variety of aid applications. Alternatively, contact your state's Department of Social Services and talk to a caseworker about your situation. A number of programs that specifically focus on pregnant women are available for low-income families, and a social worker can possibly direct you to one or more programs that will help reduce your financial burden.

Finally, make sure that your friends and family are aware of your situation and concerns. Although they may not be able support you financially, they can relieve your burden in other smaller, but valuable, ways. For instance, if you currently pay for after-school care for other children, ask friends or relatives to step in, thus eliminating the expense and worry about your children's well-being. Sometimes such small changes can make a huge difference in your emotions as well as your finances.

87. How do I cope with my other children's needs if I'm on bed rest?

This can be tricky and stressful. On one hand, you *must* prioritize your own health for the benefit of the baby you're carrying, but on the other, your children truly need your attention—you may feel torn and guilty for not being available for them.

First, let go of your guilt, as you cannot change matters. You can only do your best under difficult circumstances, and your children will survive the experience. Your pregnancy will not last forever, and soon you'll be faced with the even greater challenge of recovering from pregnancy while caring for your children *and* a new baby (and bed rest will sound like heaven!). Second, let the children know what to expect as soon as you are put on bed rest. With older children (age 10 and over), tell them truthfully about your health situation and explain why you must remain bedridden. Answer their questions and address their concerns, reassuring them that your doctors are taking care of you and that staying in bed is one way to ensure that you, and their baby brother or sister, will be fine. With younger children, avoid the nitty-gritty details—your 6-year-old will only get confused if you try to explain about an incompetent cervix or preterm labor. Let them know that your doctor told you to stay in bed so that your baby (or babies) can finish growing properly, answering any questions, concerns, or fears simply and with reassurance.

The day-to-day challenges of raising children while on prolonged bed rest can be overcome if you are willing to ask for help. Don't be afraid to ask your friends and family for assistance with child care while you're on bed rest. A friend or family member might be able to stop by even a couple hours a day—after school, for instance, when children need help with homework, or on the weekends when they're looking for something to do that's fun. Each child must spend time with you so that they don't feel that your pregnancy complications have made you *totally* inaccessible to them. Even if you only sit together and watch television, eat a meal, or talk about school, the consistency of "Mom time" will reassure the child that he or she hasn't been forgotten. The time you spend with your child or planning ways to address their needs is time that you're *not* thinking about how bored you are! Other strategies for coping with child care and stresses related to bed rest are described in Table 9 in Question 92.

88. I'm so worried about my baby's health that I'm losing sleep, and the stress is making the situation worse. What can I do?

Many times, worry and stress are related to fear of the unknown. Direct such fears to your health care staff. Ask your doctor or nurse to explain the situation very carefully and to give you an accurate estimation of your risk level. Ask for and then follow recommendations for reducing your risk level. Eat nutritious meals. Cut back on caffeine or stimulants (if you haven't already). Keep your prenatal care appointments, and above all, make a conscious effort to let go of your worries. Practice relaxation techniques that will help you sleep: Warm baths, a dinner date with your partner, regular walks in the garden, or even just a good movie at home (*not* an action film!) could be helpful. Acupuncture, shiatsu, or massage may also prove helpful if lying on a treatment table is not uncomfortable. With your doctor's permission, consider joining a yoga class—indeed, many yoga instructors have special classes designed with pregnant women in mind, emphasizing relaxation and flexibility while eliminating positions and maneuvers that are too stressful for pregnant women's joints, ligaments, and pelvic structures.

If, after doing all these things, you are still stressed and insomniac, you may be suffering from a clinical form of anxiety. Ask your health care team to refer you to a mental health professional for evaluation. At worst, you'll end up in an office talking to someone about your fears—and even if you don't go more than once, just being able to discuss your concerns with someone could be beneficial.

89. If I was previously diagnosed with depression or anxiety, are there medications I can take that are safe during pregnancy?

In clinical depression, the brain's chemistry is disordered, leading to symptoms such as fatigue or lack of energy, feelings of worthlessness or guilt, difficulty concentrating, trouble sleeping, and sometimes thoughts of death or suicide. Some of these symptoms are similar to those caused by simply being pregnant, so it may be difficult to tell whether you are simply experiencing normal pregnancy symptoms or a renewed bout of depression. Your mental health care provider and your OB/GYN should review the medication to ensure that it is effective in controlling your depression without being harmful to the fetus. If the depression is not severe, you may be able to taper off or decrease dose levels during the first trimester, when the effects on the fetus are greatest. Do not alter your medication yourself—talk to your doctor first, particularly if you have had recent depressive episodes. For most women, pregnancy does not worsen depressive symptoms, although a small percentage of women experience more episodes (or more severe depression).

Similarly, anxiety involves disordered brain chemistry and is often treated with medications. Pregnancy appears to lessen the symptoms of some anxiety disorders, such as panic disorder, in as many as 40% of women; nevertheless, in other disorders, such as obsessive compulsive disorder, symptoms may actually worsen in about 25%. Thus, how your pregnancy affects you and your treatment will depend on your specific situation. If your symptoms decrease, you might be able to reduce your medications during the pregnancy. Maintain a strong relationship with your mental health care provider throughout your pregnancy to ensure that you are receiving appropriate medication and therapy.

The good news about the medications that treat both depression and anxiety, including some selective serotonin reuptake inhibitors such as Zoloft and Prozac and many tricyclic antidepressants, is that they have fairly good safety profiles in pregnancy. Therefore, it is usually not necessary to change treatment strategies, although the dose might need to be temporarily changed.

90. Can I safely use alternative medicine such as acupuncture, herbs, or reiki to help with stress?

This depends on many factors, as pregnancy alters your body in ways that might affect the manner in which these treatments can be applied. Most such treatments, properly used, are safe, but with all of them (and particularly with herbal medicines), the changes in your body could greatly alter their effectiveness and safety. Also, some herbal preparations may cross the placental barrier, where they have unknown effects on the fetus. Some treatments may interact poorly with treatments you're receiving for another condition in your pregnancy, such as high blood pressure or gestational diabetes. In short, the safety of alternative medicine treatments in pregnancy varies according to circumstances of the pregnancy (as well as the skill and experience of the practitioner). These guidelines should help you to know whether you should proceed with an alternative treatment.

First, be sure that the practitioner you work with is skilled, experienced, and qualified to perform the treatment. Most forms of traditional healing require a license in most states. Be sure you check out the practitioner's qualifications (see the Appendix). Equally important is keeping the lines of communication open between your obstetrician and/or maternal/fetal specialist and any alternative medicine practitioner(s) you may consult. In high-risk pregnancy, your obstetrician *must* be kept informed of what other treatments you're receiving, especially when it comes to herbal preparations, so that he or she can be certain that the use of these treatments isn't interfering with or altering the effects of standard treatments. For example, if you have PIH and your herbalist offers you a tea designed to reduce stress and lower your blood pressure and your doctor gives you a medication to do the same, your blood pressure may drop *below* normal. Similarly, you should keep your alternative practitioners—acupuncturist, herbalist, and reiki provider—up-to-date on what is happening in your obstetrician's office. Changes in your physical circumstances are just as important for a non-Western, traditional healer to know as they are for your doctor.

Second, be especially cautious when it comes to any form of herbal medicine, particularly if you are buying them from health food stores. Certain herbs can be harmful in pregnancy and should be avoided altogether (see Table 8 in Question 69 for a list of potentially harmful medicinal herbs). Furthermore, herbal preparations are not regulated by the federal government, and thus, there is really no way of determining the quality or composition of their ingredients. Unless you or someone you know is preparing the medications from raw ingredients, you can't be completely sure that the packaging accurately says what's inside. You also cannot be certain that something potentially harmful isn't included in the preparation. Even if you are using self- or herbalist-prepared herbal medicines, it's generally hard to know what effects they will have on the unborn fetus, and little information is available about whether herbal medicines interact with standard over-the-counter or prescription drugs. In short, proceed with caution, and consider discontinuing their use during your pregnancy. If you've never used herbal medicines before—now is *not* the time to start, even if someone you trust recommends them!

Some alternative therapies, however, can be beneficial in a high-risk pregnancy. Acupuncture, shiatsu, reiki, and other traditional forms of healing are usually safe in pregnancy, although they do have strict guidelines as to what techniques or points should and shouldn't be used in pregnant women. These forms of therapy can be used to support the pregnancy by strengthening the body, promoting relaxation, or addressing some of the symptoms of pregnancy.

Elizabeth's comment:

I have used a number of alternative medicine treatments in the past, but when I was in the process of trying to get pregnant, I dropped the use of herbals—I didn't want to introduce unknown effects into a developing fetus, and also, I was a little embarrassed to admit to my doctors that I was using "unconventional" medications. I continued using shiatsu and acupuncture treatments, however. They certainly helped with a number of symptoms—nausea, sinus problems, fatigue, and especially high blood pressure. Even so, my acupuncturist, Nina, couldn't treat other symptoms because she'd have to use points that stimulate uterine contractions or other problematic responses. Nina was extremely careful to explain which points she could and couldn't use and why. I'd been with her for a number of years and trusted her judgment; I may not have felt the same way if I were just starting to work with someone I didn't know. The first key point is to work with someone you trust. I will give credit to my doctors: They didn't immediately scoff at the fact that I use non-Western forms of treatment, nor did they label me a New-Age fruitcake. Therefore, the second key point is to make sure that you're working with doctors who have open minds and understand that you're not just sticking pins in yourself for the fun of it!

91. Does having a high-risk pregnancy mean that I can't have a home birth or use natural childbirth methods?

Most sources discussing home birth state flatly that home birth is not an option for women involved in a high-risk pregnancy. To a certain extent, this is true but also depends on what risk factors are involved—for instance, a physically healthy 40-year-old woman who has had no complications of any kind during her pregnancy should be able to choose a home birth. Even minor complicating factors such as a history of asthma or a similar chronic condition, if they're mild and well controlled, might not be barriers to home birth. However, most women who fall in the high-risk category because of significant health problems are better advised to give birth in a hospital or a birthing center affiliated with a hospital so that emergency medical care is available. If you are considering home birth, talk to your doctor about the potential risks of home birth in your situation.

Giving birth in a hospital or birthing center does not mean that you must give up on natural childbirth methods, however. In fact, many hospitals encourage laboring mothers to make use of such techniques, as they limit the use of medications during labor. If natural childbirth is important to you, discuss the matter with your obstetrician *before* you arrive at the hospital. Most hospitals offer the opportunity to submit a birth plan in advance—so take the time to sit down and work one out; having the details of what you do and don't want while you're in labor can be very helpful information. Unless your pregnancy is severely complicated with a potential for labor complications or if there's a need for specialized postpartum care, your birth plan will likely be acceptable, although many labor experiences do not go as envisioned by the prospective mother! Visit the hospital's labor and delivery rooms or birth center before your due date to see the facilities, and don't be afraid to ask for a tour.

92. Being on bed rest week after week is driving me crazy. I'm so bored and lonely lying here all day. Can I do something to pass the time without harming myself or the baby?

Mothers—particularly working mothers—tend to have a love–hate relationship with bed rest. On one hand, the mother on bed rest can spend all her time "lounging," guilt-free, on "doctor's orders," but on the other, after about week, the mom to be is ready to climb the walls with boredom. Nevertheless, she is afraid to ignore her doctor's instructions for fear of harming her baby, in some cases with good reason. Bed rest seems like a vacation only to those who've never been on it!

The strategies listed in Table 9 can help you to cope with bed rest. Keep in touch with friends, family, and colleagues via phone, e-mail, instant messaging, or even good, old-fashioned paper letters, but don't let yourself become isolated.

Table 9   Coping with Bed Rest

Daily routine:

Being bored is one of the hardest aspects of bed rest. Getting yourself through each day can be a tough challenge. Here are some suggestions:

- Know that you are not alone. Many other women are struggling through bed rest right now!!
- Try to keep a positive attitude. It is hard, but it helps.
- Read one of the books or magazines on pregnancy bed rest. They are full of good ideas and things you will need to know.
- If you are on home bed rest, set up an efficient place to rest close to a bathroom. Try to be close to a window. Have tables nearby, a telephone, television with VCR if possible, computer, writing materials, and books. Keep a cooler or small refrigerator by your bed or couch. Fill it with juice, meals, and snacks for the day. You need to drink plenty of fluids. Plan to drink 8 ounces an hour while you are awake (soda and coffee do not count because they dehydrate you).
- Change into regular clothes each morning and put pajamas on at night to keep your days and nights separate. Try spending the day in one room and sleep at night in another room if possible.
- Get yourself on a schedule. Time will pass more quickly if you establish a routine for yourself.
- Since you cannot do the usual household responsibilities, try to do other activities like paying the bills, balancing the checkbook, making grocery lists, and organizing other people to help with other chores.
- At first you may feel like you shouldn't bother people, but it is very important to let other people help out. It will relieve the stress on you and your family, so take advantage of any offers from family, friends, church members, neighbors, coworkers, (and anyone else!), to help with childcare, housework, walking the dog, shoveling snow, errands, or just keeping you company.
- Make lists of baby things, including baby names, things you will need for the baby like clothes, furniture, nursery supplies, and all the other baby equipment.
- Organize photos into albums, rearrange sock drawers or any junk drawers in the house, write letters, read books, talk on the phone, try sewing, knitting, needlepoint, latch hook or any other crafts, anything to keep your mind occupied and stimulated.
- Keep a journal of your thoughts and frustrations, or of thoughts, feelings and hopes about your baby.
- Most importantly, talk to other women who have been on bed rest. Nobody knows what it is like unless you have been there. Contact Sidelines (see Appendix) to find out more about talking with other women as well as other benefits. Read online bulletin boards for other messages from women on bed rest.

Getting along with partner:

Bed rest is very difficult for families. Concern about the baby and overwhelming responsibilities can take a toll on any relationship. It is important to try

(continued)

Table 9 Continued

to keep open and supportive communication between you and your partner. You both may feel isolated and frustrated, and cannot fully know what the other is experiencing. You would love to have more to do and your partner would love to have less to do, so sometimes you have very different feelings. Incorporate a daily time set aside for each of you to vent and hear what the other is going through. Order takeout food from your favorite restaurant, or watch a movie together. If things get more serious and you are unable to talk to each other, talk to a therapist, counselor, or minister to help you work through some of these difficulties.

Financial concerns:

Many families have financial problems as a result of bed rest. Often times the woman's income is partially or completely lost. Even if medical bills are covered by insurance, loss of income and extra costs are concerning to families. Many women take their "maternity leave" and vacation and sick time during a high-risk pregnancy. But often this does not last long enough, and sometimes women find they can't go back to work right away after the baby is born. Financial concerns can add stress and increase marital tension. Find a financial counselor to help manage financial disruption.

Child care management:

Care for other children while their mother is on bed rest is a major challenge for many families. This often contributes to the financial crisis of bed rest. Children of any age become upset when their mother is absent, and mothers worry about the disrupted routines and inconsistencies her children face. Rather than trying to find short-term day care, try to make long-term child care arrangements to provide stability for the children. It will also be much more stressful for you and your partner to try to find child care for each day. So plan for the long term and cancel plans if you don't end up needing it that long. Some important things to remember about child care are:

- Care should be as consistent as possible so that the child will feel secure
- Give the child a positive reason why you can't get up or come home from the hospital
- Children often worry when things go wrong and are different. Sometimes they think they are the cause of things, therefore you should avoid telling a young child that "mommy is sick." It may be better to say something like, "I have to stay in bed so that the baby can be healthy when it is born"
- Find some "quiet time" each day to spend with your child if you can. Watch a video or take a nap together, sing, cut and paste pictures, etc. You both need this time together and will feel better.
- Try to have your child do active play before the quiet time so he/she is not so restless.

SOURCE: Pregnancy Bed Rest: Frequently Asked Questions. Available at http://fpb.cwru.edu/Bedrest/FAQ/daytoday.shtm (accessed January 11, 2008). Used with permission from Judy Maloni, PhD, RN, FAAN, Nursing Professor and Pregnancy Bed Rest Researcher, Case Western Reserve University, Bolton School of Nursing. © Case Western Reserve University, 2005.

Elizabeth's comment:

I've got two recommendations for women on bed rest: first, get yourself a buddy, someone who will check in with you a couple of times a day by phone—just so you have someone to talk to. An organization called Sidelines pairs women on bed rest with "buddy" volunteers (see the Appendix). Second, let all of your friends and relatives know that you need books, movies, and CDs to eliminate boredom. I read or re-read every book I owned during the first week and by the second week had gone through all of the books given to me by friends and relatives. Daytime television was appalling, and I nearly went berserk with boredom. My sanity was saved by joining Netflix: I used to pray for the arrival of those red envelopes with new movies. It was unquestionably the longest 4 weeks of my entire life. I got through it by keeping my "eyes on the prize": I wanted a healthy, full-term baby, which is what I got.

93. What do I do if I have no health insurance to pay for all of the medical tests and procedures?

If you have no health insurance or only minimal coverage, talk to your doctor; he or she can likely direct you to a caseworker who can help you handle this situation. Health insurance plans that are specifically geared toward pregnant women are available. Some of these can be found online through organizations focused on pregnancy (see the Appendix). If your income is too low to afford conventional insurance, then you might be eligible for Medicaid assistance. In most states, the cutoff level is around $30,000 in annual income, but the guidelines for Medicaid enrollment vary from state to state. Contact your state's Department of Health and Human Services (or equivalent) to ask about eligibility. You may be able to get help in applying for benefits from the hospital or clinic where you're receiving prenatal care, as most institutions have caseworkers who are skilled in navigating insurance and government assistance programs.

94. Are support groups or health professionals available for women during a high-risk pregnancy?

As high-risk pregnancy has become more common, organizations targeting the needs of high-risk mothers have appeared. Many of these are easily accessed online, which is terrific if you have Internet access but unfortunate if you don't. Some, however, can be reached through conventional means, and at least one—the March of Dimes—has had long-term experience in addressing the needs of women undergoing high-risk pregnancy, particularly those pregnancies associated with birth defects. A listing of Web sites and organizations offering support to pregnant women is found in the Appendix under the "Support Groups" heading.

Most of your health needs in high-risk pregnancy can be appropriately served by any competent OB/GYN physician or nurse. However, you may need the care of a maternal/fetal specialist (also known as a perinatologist). If your own doctor cannot provide a referral, then contact one of several organizations that provide listings of maternal/fetal specialists in the United States. These organizations are listed in the Appendix under the "Specialist Listings" heading.

PART NINE

Facing Loss in High-Risk Pregnancy

I've already lost two pregnancies, and I'm terrified of losing this one. Can I do anything to lower my risk of another miscarriage?

I'm at high risk for preterm labor and am worried about the harm early delivery could do to my baby. How early is too early? What are the baby's chances of survival if he or she comes early?

What causes a baby to be stillborn? Is there some way to prevent stillbirth?

More . . .

95. I've already lost two pregnancies, and I'm terrified of losing this one. Can I do anything to lower my risk of another miscarriage?

Losing one pregnancy to miscarriage is usually just happenstance. Losing two could also just be coincidence—but it may mean there's an underlying health issue. Your doctor will likely monitor your pregnancy closely from the outset to watch for problems, but unless a specific issue is identified, he or she cannot do much medically to help you avoid another. Nevertheless, here are some things you can do to lessen your risk of miscarriage:

Eliminate caffeine. Recent data indicate that drinking caffeinated beverages—up to five cups of coffee daily or the equivalent—can double the incidence of miscarriage. Caffeine can cause dehydration and also raise your blood pressure and dilate (close) your blood vessels—any or all of which might contribute to miscarriage. If you have a caffeine habit, break it; your chances of avoiding a miscarriage will improve if you do. You will likely experience some withdrawal symptoms such as headaches, so discuss the situation with your doctor before you start—it may be better to lower your intake gradually rather than all at once, depending on how much you drink each day. Also, make sure that you replace the coffee, tea, or cola with water, juice, or milk, rather than just switching to decaf. Any of these beverages will hydrate you effectively and provide nutritional support.

Be proactive: Consult a maternal/fetal medicine specialist early on to look for "fixable" factors.

Practice healthy living. Get at least 8 hours of sleep each night (and naps if you become fatigued). Eat a balanced diet. Take your prenatal vitamin each day. Be sure to exercise. Stay hydrated, and avoid junk food, cigarettes, alcohol, and recreational drugs. The better you treat your body, the better it will treat you.

Be proactive. Particularly if you've ever had a miscarriage after 10 weeks, you may want to consult a maternal/fetal medicine specialist early on to look for "fixable" factors. Some women with unidentified **thrombophilias**—factors causing blood to clot more readily—are at risk for miscarriage, preeclampsia, intrauterine growth restriction, and placental abruption. If you ever stopped using birth control pills because of clotting concerns, thrombophilia may be part of the problem. This can be controlled by using heparin, an anticlotting agent. Uterine abnormalities, unidentified infections of the cervix or uterus, and other factors can also be identified and corrected to lower your risk of miscarriage.

Thrombophilias
Factors that cause blood to clot more readily.

De-stress. Don't let your worries, particularly about miscarriage, overwhelm you. Practice relaxation techniques, or find ways to distract yourself from concerns. Better still, save them for your doctor's visits, where you can express them and receive honest, direct answers. Talk to a therapist, a minister, or a close friend. Look for online support groups (see the Appendix). If alternative medicine interests you, visit an acupuncturist, shiatsu therapist, or reiki provider—often, such treatments focus on emotional and physical relaxation. Release your fears in whatever way suits you best.

Following these instructions exactly will not necessarily eliminate miscarriage. The causes of miscarriage are usually complex and without apparent reason. Still, it will help if you make an effort to be as healthy as possible during your pregnancy, and hope for the best (see Question 99 for more on this subject).

96. I'm at high risk for preterm labor and am worried about the harm early delivery could do to my baby. How early is too early? What are the baby's chances of survival if he or she comes early?

The duration of a pregnancy is 40 weeks from the date of the mother's last menstrual period, but a fetus is considered full term at 37 weeks. Generally, the baby will suffer few or no ill

Respiratory distress syndrome (RDS)

Poor lung function in premature infants that is often caused by lack of surfactant in the lungs.

Necrotizing enterocolitis

A gastrointestinal disease, usually affecting premature infants, in which infection and inflammation damage the intestine.

effects if delivered at 35 weeks or later. A fetus delivered prior to 35 weeks, however, may suffer health effects such as **respiratory distress syndrome (RDS),** bleeding in the brain, and an intestinal inflammation called **necrotizing enterocolitis.** The earlier the delivery, the greater are the risks of adverse effects, including the possibility that the baby might not survive. Currently, a baby's chance of survival at 24 weeks is about 50% to 60%, about 70% at 25 weeks, 80% from 26 to 28 weeks, and 90% at 28 to 32 weeks. There is no difference from that of full-term babies after about 32 weeks. Survival can also vary depending on the baby's gender (girls tend to do better than boys), whether more than one fetus is involved (singletons do better than multiples), and whether a corticosteroid called betamethasone, which can prevent brain bleeding and help lung function, was administered before delivery. The record for survival for a premature baby is currently 21 weeks 6 days, but it is extraordinarily rare for a baby under 24 weeks to survive. Whether doctors should even attempt to save such tiny infants given the negative health effects of extremely premature babies is controversial.

Very early deliveries, 32 weeks or less, may mean that the child will suffer long-term physical effects such as vision problems or blindness, breathing disorders, difficulty digesting food, and sometimes brain damage or mental handicaps (see Question 84). Survival means that the baby is alive, not that he or she is healthy, although some very early preemies go on to become completely normal, healthy children. As intervention methods become more sophisticated, preemies of younger gestational age are surviving more often, and treatments are improving.

Unquestionably, the likelihood of survival for a severely premature baby is helped by (1) the mother having good overall health and proper prenatal care before preterm labor begins and (2) the use of corticosteroid medications prior to birth (see Question 82). Both of these factors contribute to improved physical development in the fetus, particularly in its ability to breathe.

97. What causes a baby to be stillborn? Is there some way to prevent stillbirth?

Stillbirth is defined as the death of the fetus after 20 weeks of pregnancy. The causes are varied: placental or umbilical blood flow problems, birth defects, infections, maternal health problems, use of tobacco, drugs, or alcohol during pregnancy. Any of these can contribute to stillbirth. Sometimes death occurs during labor because of an unforeseen complication, such as umbilical cord prolapse.

Some steps can be taken to reduce your risk of stillbirth. Take good care of your own health, and work closely with your prenatal care providers. Regular prenatal appointments help to pinpoint any concerns before they fully develop and may permit your doctor to intervene before the problem becomes life threatening for the baby. Taking care of your health also means avoiding sources of infection (such as those listed in Question 29) and immediately reporting any unusual symptoms, especially pain or bleeding, to your doctor. In addition, after about 26 weeks, monitor your baby's movements to get a sense of his or her normal level of activity. Knowing what's normal is important in determining whether the baby's activity is unusually low or high, which can be the first indication of distress.

98. I've been told that my baby has a life-threatening condition and probably won't survive after birth. How do I cope with this information?

A diagnosis of a fatal illness in an unborn child is perhaps the most difficult situation an expectant parent can face. Several critical steps can be taken to help you and your partner cope with this situation.

Get a second opinion. Although you may have the best obstetrician or maternal/fetal medicine specialist in the city, the country, the continent, or the universe, he or she is still not infallible. A second opinion will confirm whether your doctor's diagnosis is accurate, enabling you to prepare yourself for the eventual loss of your child. Few doctors will have any difficulty offering you a referral in such cases. Our own policy is to encourage second opinions, and we routinely provide referrals even if the parents don't ask for one.

Rally your emotional support. Many people feel that they need to be "brave" or "show grace under pressure" by keeping the diagnosis private and refusing to show their emotional upset. Tell your relatives and friends what is going on, and let them know that you need them. Explore the possibility of having regular sessions with a grief counselor, even before the baby's birth.

Live in the moment. Your time with your unborn child will be short—this is something you already know. What you do not know—what nobody knows, even your doctor—is *how much* time you will have with this child. Therefore, you will likely find greater comfort after his or her death if you make the most of the time you have while the child is still with you, even before birth. Children do show personality traits while in the womb, and after a certain stage of development, they can even hear what goes on outside. You and your partner should talk and interact with your child, even before birth. Give the child a name so that he or she has a distinct identity. Why do this? If the baby already has a personal history before death, you will have more to celebrate and hold on to when the time comes to let the child go.

Because there is no certainty about how long the baby will live after birth—some children with severe, fatal conditions nonetheless live for weeks, months, or even years—you may wish to consider planning a small, traditional celebration such as a christening, a bris, or a home-from-hospital party for the first few days after the child's birth. Although the celebrations may have sad undertones, they will nonetheless be important markers of the brief time that you had with your child.

Prepare yourself. Part of living in the moment is being aware of the future. As discussed in Question 99, there are ways to grieve that honor your child and help you recover from the loss.

99. If I lose my baby, how will I ever be able to recover?

Coping with the loss of a pregnancy is one of the most difficult, emotionally wrenching circumstances any parent can face. How you will cope with it depends largely on your own skills in handling loss, your sources of emotional support, and your willingness to look for resources to help you through this crisis. The situation may be all the more acute if this is your first child, if your relationship with the baby's other parent isn't strong or close, if you have never experienced the death of a relative or loved one, or if you lack a strong network of friends. Everyone's experiences in this regard differ, so there is no one-size-fits-all method to grief. You will experience whatever is appropriate for you, and it will differ from what other people experience.

However, although the subjects of miscarriages or the death of an unborn child are not often discussed, even among close friends, loss in pregnancy is fairly common. Raising the issue with other women friends will undoubtedly turn up one or two (or more!) who also have experienced this tragedy—sometimes more than once. It is particularly difficult emotionally if this is a first child, an unintended pregnancy, or a child to whom much emotional baggage is attached (a first grandchild, the long-awaited result of infertility treatments, and so on). You might wonder what you have done to deserve this, or you might experience feelings of guilt or inadequacy. Other people for whom this child had strong emotional significance may also be disappointed and thus encourage your guilty feelings. If you have never been told that miscarriages happen for many reasons, you may tend to believe these people, particularly while you are so vulnerable from the emotional, mood, and hormone swings—*but you should not.* **Don't** listen to people who state or imply that you did something to cause your miscarriage. Usually, the cause of the miscarriage stems from an inherent problem in the fetus. It has *nothing whatsoever* to do with anything you did, ate, drank, thought, felt, or prayed for. A slip off an icy step or overexertion moving furniture around wasn't the culprit, either. Generally, it isn't that easy to lose a healthy pregnancy. Miscarriage is often Nature's way of removing a pregnancy that would not or could not produce a viable, living child. Conversely, many physiological cushions protect an unborn fetus from trauma; thus, if the pregnancy itself is healthy and viable, chances are good that no mere accident can end it. Again, *you did nothing to cause this loss.*

Most of the time, miscarriage has nothing whatsoever to do with anything you did, ate, drank, thought, felt, or prayed for.

Because this child probably had a tentative name and may have developed a "personality," you might find it helpful to have a memorial event. You might want to have a religious service that provides an ending and a place for remembrance. This service might include a statement of hope for the renewed health of the family, a few words about the positive experiences that you had during pregnancy, and permission to say goodbye in some way that is appropriate. A burial service and perhaps a request for baptism, although unusual, may also help you feel that your child is part of the community that you belong to. If you are not a religious person, you still might find comfort in planting a garden with a special tree or perhaps by volunteering or making a donation to an organization that supports children in need. You must understand that you have a right to grieve and that you should express it in whatever way gives you solace. In our experience, parents should not to try to pretend that a miscarriage or stillbirth is not the loss of a person or a member of their family, even if the loss occurs early in the pregnancy. Our patients typically form an emotional attachment to the fetus when they see the ultrasound image. Thus, you should allow yourself and your partner to grieve just as you would for any other family member who died.

Some may say, "You can always have another baby." They do not mean to be unkind; their statement simply minimizes their awareness that the loss of a child, even one still unborn, is a very painful event. You may feel helpless if you have no real answer, medical or otherwise, about why this loss occurred. Only the people who have had a similar experience will truly understand. Explore options for support groups offered at some hospitals. Your doctor should schedule a follow-up visit so that he or she can help you process the loss and make sense of what went wrong; if possible, try to go with your partner or a supportive friend or family member. You had expected to go back to see your doctor with a new baby; the pregnancy was connected emotionally to these visits, and some extra support can be beneficial.

Understand that you *will* get past this tragedy. Not that it will ever leave you, but at some point, your life will resume a pattern of normalcy. You will work and play. You will resume your life with your spouse or partner. Perhaps someday you will get pregnant again . . . or you may not. However, you cannot remain stuck on this event. If you are, then you may be suffering from depression and should seek professional help from a therapist or a clergyperson. The death of a child, even an unborn one, can be all-consuming, but sooner or later, your life, although greatly changed, will continue.

Elizabeth's comment:

I was fortunate that I didn't lose either of my sons, but I know many women who have lost babies. All of my immediate female relatives have lost at least one pregnancy. I've seen friends lose babies as late as 6 months into the pregnancy. This is heart wrenching. The only lesson I can take from watching them is this: Acknowledge the loss, honor your grief, and do what you can to get through. Then one day, you will find that it's behind you. It is never completely in your past—more than 40 years afterward, my aunt still recalls the baby she lost that would have been my age—but it eventually is no longer the focus of your day-to-day life. You mourn, just as you would mourn someone you'd known all your life, and then you move on in the same way as you do after the death of any loved one.

100. Where can I go for more information about high-risk pregnancy?

The Appendix contains a number of resources that address high-risk pregnancy generally and specifically. We encourage you to use them in conjunction with the information you get from your doctor to help manage your current or future pregnancies.

Appendix

The following are resources we have found to be valuable for patients. Each entry has been reviewed to make sure that the Web site is active and links to the correct page, but we make no claims as to the value of the information you will find on these Web sites. For specific resources, we have put a few comments after each listing to describe what you will find; where the comments are in quotes, they have been derived directly from the site's "About Us" information. Many of the sites listed here have links to other sites that may be valuable to you.

General High-Risk Pregnancy Information Online

The American College of Obstetrics and Gynecology
www.acog.org

The American Pregnancy Association
www.americanpregnancy.org

The Centers for Disease Control and Prevention
www.cdc.gov/ncbddd/pregnancy_gateway/now.htm

National Institutes of Health
www.nlm.nih.gov/medlineplus/highriskpregnancy.html

The Merck Manuals Online Medical Library
www.merck.com/mmhe/sec22/ch258/ch258a.html

OBFocus High Risk Pregnancy Directory
www.obfocus.com

University of Virginia High-Risk Pregnancy Site
www.healthsystem.virginia.edu/uvahealth/peds_hrpregnant/index.cfm

Bed Rest

Case Western Reserve University/Judith Maloni, PhD, RN, FAAN
Pregnancy Bed Rest: Information and Support for Families and Caregivers
http://fpb.cwru.edu/Bedrest/
Comprehensive site devoted to issues related to pregnancy bed rest—one of the most complete sources of information out there.

Birth Defects
Organizations that sponsor research on and parental assistance for specific birth defects are listed here. These listings represent a small subsample of the many organizations out there for various birth defects and pregnancy-related disorders.

Cystic Fibrosis Foundation
National headquarters:
6931 Arlington Road
Bethesda, MD 20814
Phone: 1-301-951-4422
Toll free: 1-800-FIGHT CF (344-4823)
E-mail: info@cff.org (see the chapter directory for local e-mail addresses)
Fax: 1-301-951-6378
Web site: *www.cff.org*
"The mission of the Cystic Fibrosis Foundation, a nonprofit, donor-supported organization, is to assure the development of the means to cure and control cystic fibrosis and to improve the quality of life for those with the disease."

The March of Dimes
(see listing under *Premature/Special Needs Infants*)

National Center on Birth Defects and Developmental Disabilities (NCBDDD)
Centers for Disease Control and Prevention
1600 Clifton Road
Atlanta, GA 30333
Phone: 1-800-CDC-INFO (232-4636); 1-888-232-6348 (TTY)
Web site: *www.cdc.gov/ncbddd/default.htm*
Provides basic information about a great many different birth defects, both physical and developmental. An excellent starting point for research on specific birth defects.

National Down Syndrome Society
666 Broadway
New York, NY 10012
E-mail: info@ndss.org
Phone: 1-800-221-4602
Fax: 1-212-979-2873
Web site: *www.ndss.org*
"The National Down Syndrome Society envisions a world in which all people with Down syndrome have the opportunity to realize their life aspirations. NDSS is committed to being the national leader in enhancing the quality of life, and realizing the potential of all people with Down syndrome. The mission of the National Down Syndrome Society is to benefit people with Down syndrome and their families through national leadership in education, research and advocacy."

Osteogenesis Imperfecta Foundation
804 W. Diamond Avenue, Suite 210
Gaithersburg, MD 20878
Phone: 1-800-981-2663 or 1-301-947-0083
Fax: 1-301-947-0456
Web site: *www.oif.org*
E-mail: bonelink@oif.org
"The Osteogenesis Imperfecta Foundation, Inc. (OI Foundation) is the only voluntary national health organization dedicated to helping people cope with the problems associated with osteogenesis imperfecta. The Foundation's mission is to improve the quality of life for people affected by OI through research to find treatments and a cure, education, awareness, and mutual support."

Complementary and Alternative Medicine (CAM)

Acupuncture Today
Corporate Office
PO Box 4139
Huntington Beach, CA 92605-4139
Phone: 1-714-230-3150
Fax: 1-714-899-4273
Web site: *www.acupuncturetoday.com*
Offers information about how acupuncture is used to treat a variety of conditions.

Appendix

National Center for Complementary and Alternative Medicine Clearinghouse
Toll-free in the United States: 1-888-644-6226
TTY (for deaf and hard-of-hearing callers): 1-866-464-3615
Web site: *www.nccam.nih.gov*
E-mail: info@nccam.nih.gov
"The NCCAM Clearinghouse provides information on CAM and NCCAM, including publications and searches of Federal databases of scientific and medical literature. The Clearinghouse does not provide medical advice, treatment recommendations, or referrals to practitioners."

National Certification Commission for Acupuncture and Oriental Medicine
76 South Laura Street Suite 1290
Jacksonville, FL 32202
Phone: 1-904-598-1005
Fax: 1-904-598-5001
Web site: *www.nccaom.org*
"The National Certification Commission for Acupuncture and Oriental Medicine (NCCAOM) is a non-profit organization established in 1982. It currently operates under Section 501(c)(6) of the Internal Revenue code. Its mission is to establish, assess, and promote recognized standards of competence and safety in acupuncture and Oriental medicine for the protection and benefit of the public."

Employment

U.S. Equal Employment Opportunity Commission
Headquarters:
1801 L Street N.W.
Washington, DC 20507
Phone: 1-202-663-4900
TTY: 1-202-663-4494
National:
Phone: 1-800-669-4000; TTY number is 1-800-669-6820
E-mail: info@eeoc.gov (please include your zip code and/or city and state so that your e-mail will be sent to the appropriate office)
Pregnancy Discrimination Act information: *http://www.eeoc.gov/types/pregnancy.html*
Complaints: *http://www.eeoc.gov/facts/howtofil.html*
Contacting the EEOC: There are local and regional offices throughout the United States. You should contact the office nearest you. EEOC representatives are available

to assist you between 8:30 a.m. and 5:30 p.m. Eastern Time. An automated system with answers to frequently asked questions is available on a 24-hour basis.

Fetal Alcohol Spectrum Disorder/Fetal Alcohol Syndrome

FASD Center for Excellence
Substance and Mental Health Services Administration
Department of Health and Human Services
2101 Gaither Road, Suite 600
Rockville, MD 20850
Phone: 1-866-STOPFAS (786-7327)
Web site: *www.fasdcenter.samhsa.gov*
E-mail: patricia.getty@samhsa.hhs.gov

Fish Advisories

U.S. Environmental Protection Agency
Fish Advisory Program
Office of Science and Technology (4303T)
1200 Pennsylvania Avenue N.W.
Washington, DC 20460
or call the Standards and Health Protection Division at 1-202-566-0400
Web site: *www.epa.gov/waterscience/fish/*
Links to local fish advisory programs can be found at *www.epa.gov/waterscience/fish/states.htm*

Gestational Diabetes

American Diabetes Association
ATTN: National Call Center
1701 North Beauregard Street
Alexandria, VA 22311
Phone: 1-800-DIABETES (1-800-342-2383)
Web site: *www.diabetes.org*
A resource offering useful information about diabetes management in general and gestational diabetes in particular. Nutrition, exercise, and prevention are topics of particular interest.

Herbal/Natural Medicines

NIH Medline Plus
www.nlm.nih.gov/medlineplus/druginformation.html

Natural Medicines Database
www.naturaldatabase.com

Natural Standard
245 First Street, 18th Floor
Cambridge, MA 02142
Phone: 1-617-444-8629
Web site: www.naturalstandard.com
"Natural Standard is an international research collaboration that aggregates and synthesizes data on complementary and alternative therapies. Using a comprehensive methodology and reproducible grading scales, information is created that is evidence-based, consensus-based, and peer-reviewed, tapping into the collective expertise of a multidisciplinary Editorial Board. The mission of this collaboration is to provide objective, reliable information that aids clinicians, patients, and healthcare institutions to make more informed and safer therapeutic decisions."

Hypertension, see PIH/Preeclampsia

Miscarriage/Pregnancy Loss

American Pregnancy Association
Visit Web site or write to them for information about miscarriage (*see* General Information Online *or look under* Specialist Listings *for contact info*)

FertilityPlus
www.fertilityplus.org/faq/miscarriage/resources.html
FertilityPlus is a nonprofit Web site for patient information on trying to conceive that includes information on miscarriage and helpful links. Information is written by patients for patients.

PIH/Preeclampsia

Preeclampsia Foundation
5353 Wayzata Boulevard, Suite 207
Minneapolis, MN 55416
Phone: 1-800-665-9341
Toll Free: 1-952-252-3573
Phone: 1-952-252-8096
E-mail: info@preeclampsia.org
Web site: *www.preeclampsia.org*
"Preeclampsia Foundation is a 501 (c) (3) non-profit operating organization established in the year 2000 to promote safe pregnancy and postpartum research, public education and patient support. The Preeclampsia Foundation's mission is to reduce maternal and infant illness and death due to preeclampsia by supporting innovative research, raising public awareness, and helping women access safe reproductive technology, support and care."

Premature/Special Needs Infants
(*See also* Birth Defects *for organizations that investigate and support specific defects.*)

March of Dimes
National Office
1275 Mamaroneck Avenue
White Plains, NY 10605
Phone: 1-914-997-4488
Web site: *www.marchofdimes.com*
March of Dimes is dedicated to improving the health of babies by preventing birth defects, premature birth, and infant mortality. It carries out this mission through research, community services, education, and advocacy. One particularly helpful program offered by the March of Dimes supports parents whose babies are in NICUs. Individual chapters in each state may be contacted for assistance by parents with premature or special needs infants.

Prematurity

www.prematurity.org

"Prematurity is a volunteer preemie website from our family for your preemie. Our goal is to support preemie parents by providing information on prematurity and preemie care. Since 1996, the Prematurity website has been a top ranked preemie support site in major search engines, preemie books, TV, and the news. Preemie Child, our support group for parents of school age preemies, is the first and only major preemie parent organization for the growing population of older preemies."

PUPPP Relief

Naomi's PUPPP Page

http://www.tcinternet.net/users/kritzerburke/naomi/PUPPP.htm

This is an excellent description of what PUPPP is and the many remedies, effective and otherwise, that are available for it. It is a must read if you have PUPPP, and it includes a number of useful links.

Rainier Soapworks

13501 103rd Avenue East

Puyallup, WA 98374-3004

Web site: *www.rainiersoapworks.com*

This company makes natural soaps and herbal creams for a variety of skin problems, including PUPPP. One author (Elizabeth) has tried them with some success. This does not mean they work for everyone, but it's a starting point.

Grandpa Brands Company

1820 Airport Exchange Boulevard

Erlanger, KY 41018

Phone: 1-800-684-1468 or 1-859-647-0777

Fax: 1-859-647-0778

E-mail: kimberly@grandpabrands.com

They are makers of pine tar soap and shampoo, which is very effective for itchy rashes of all kinds.

Smoking Cessation

Smokefree.gov is an online resource for people who want to stop smoking, sponsored by the federal government. Alternatively, smokers may call the toll-free number 1-800-QUIT-NOW.

The **Tobacco Research and Intervention Program (TRIP)** helps women who are pregnant and who have quit smoking to remain smoke free. For an informational booklet about staying smoke free, call this toll-free number: 1-877-954-2548.

The **American College of Obstetricians and Gynecologists** provides information for health care providers to assist them as they help patients stop smoking (see full listing under *General High-Risk Pregnancy Information Online*).

Specialist Listings

Each of the organizations listed below has a Web site that includes an online physician locator form that can be used to request listings of specialists in your area.

American College of Obstetricians and Gynecologists
409 12th Street S.W., PO Box 96920
Washington, DC 20090-6920
Phone: 1-202-638-5577
Physician directory online: *www.acog.org/member-lookup/disclaimer.cfm*

American Pregnancy Association
1425 Greenway Drive, Suite 440
Irving, Texas 75038
Phone: 1-972-550-0140
Fax: 1-972-550-0800
E-mail: Questions@AmericanPregnancy.org
Web site: *www.americanpregnancy.org*

Society for Maternal-Fetal Medicine
409 12th Street SW
Washington, DC 20024
Phone: 1-202-863-2476
Fax: 1-202-554-1132
E-mail: smfm@smfm.org
Web site: *www.smfm.org*

Sidelines National Support Network (see full listing under *Support Groups*)
www.sidelines.org

Support Groups

Empty Cradles
www.empty-cradles.com
A Web site devoted to support of parents who have lost a baby due to miscarriage, stillbirth, SIDS, and so on; includes chat rooms and articles on several related topics.

March of Dimes (see full listing under *Premature/Special Needs Infants***)**
www.marchofdimes.com

Sidelines National Support Network
PO Box 1808
Laguna Beach, CA 92652
Phone: 1-888-447-4754
Fax: 1-949-497-5598
E-mail address for National Office: sidelines@sidelines.org
Web site: *www.sidelines.org*
Sidelines is a 501 (c)(3) nonprofit organization providing international support for women and their families experiencing complicated pregnancies and premature births. Their mission is to help families cope more successfully with a high-risk pregnancy with appropriate medical intervention, education, and a strong support system.

Glossary

A

Addiction: Inability to control or stop the use of alcohol, tobacco, illegal drugs, or prescription medications.

Amniocentesis: Collection of fetal cells using a needle guided into the amniotic sac.

Anemia: Low red blood cell count.

Anorexia: An eating disorder in which poor body image impairs the ability to eat, leading to gradual starvation.

Apgar scores: A series of tests after delivery that identify babies who have trouble adjusting to the outside environment.

Areola: The circle of dark, sensitive skin surrounding the nipple of each breast.

Asymptomatic genetic carrier: A person who, having inherited a defective gene from one parent, shows no symptoms of illness but can pass the disease to his or her children.

Autoimmune disorder: A disorder in which the immune system attacks the body's own cells.

Autosomal dominant disease: An inherited disorder in which only one defective gene is required for the disease to occur.

Autosomal recessive disease: An inherited disorder in which a defective gene from each parent is required for the disease to occur.

B

Back labor: Labor in which the baby is positioned facing up rather than down.

Baseline: The starting point; in medicine, the normal values for a given person.

Bed rest: A prescription requiring a patient to rest in bed part or all of the day as well as night.

Benign: Causing no or little harm.

Bilirubin: A substance produced by the spleen that can be elevated in certain diseases.

Biophysical age: Physical condition in comparison to the expected standard for the number of years one has lived.

Biophysical profile: A collection of measurements taken by ultrasound that assess the baby's health and growth rate.

Blastocyst: Early stage of a fertilized egg in which the egg divides and forms a hollow ball before implantation in the uterus.

Braxton-Hicks contractions: Contractions occurring before labor that function as "practice" for the uterus.

Breech birth: Birth in which the baby is not head down in the birth canal but is positioned feet or buttocks first.

Bulimia: An eating disorder characterized by alternating cycles of binge eating and purging (vomiting).

C

Carbohydrates: Simple and complex sugars and starches in food.

Carbon monoxide: A toxin found in cigarette smoke and car exhaust.

Cerclage: A procedure in which the cervix is stitched shut to prevent premature opening.

Cesarean section: Surgery to extract the fetus from the uterus through the abdomen when vaginal birth is not possible or dangerous.

Chorionic villus sampling: Collection of fetal cells from the uterus for diagnosis of chromosomal disorders.

Chronic: Long-term, ongoing disorders or conditions.

Complete bed rest: Bed rest in which the mother is forbidden to arise from bed for any reason.

Complete blood count (CBC): An analysis of the various blood cells to determine whether any blood-related health issues are present.

Congenital: Present before birth.

Congenital diaphragmatic hernia: A birth defect in which the liver is located in the chest, causing the lungs to be compressed and poorly developed.

Conjoined twins: Twins that fail to separate during development of the embryos.

Cord prolapse: A situation in which the umbilical cord slips out of the uterus in advance of the baby, potentially interfering with the baby's blood supply.

Cord stricture: Constriction or blockage of the umbilical cord.

Corticosteroid medications: Medications that can induce production of surfactant in a preterm fetus.

Corticotrophin-releasing hormone: A hormone released by the placenta near the end of the pregnancy to stimulate changes that precede delivery.

Cortisol: An adrenal gland hormone.

Cytomegalovirus (CMV): A virus generally harmless to adults or children, but dangerous to unborn babies.

D

Dehydration: Insufficient water intake, leading to too little fluid in the body.

Diabetes: A condition in which the body lacks the ability to produce or use insulin to convert the glucose into energy.

Diastolic: Blood pressure during the resting phase of the heartbeat.

Diuretic: Causing increased urination and fluid loss.

Down syndrome: A chromosomal abnormality (trisomy 21) that leads to variable levels of mental retardation and physical defects.

E

Eclampsia: Severe hypertension in pregnancy characterized by seizures and coma.

Edema: Swelling caused by collection of fluid under the skin.

Edwards syndrome: A chromosomal abnormality (trisomy 18) causing severe physical defects that is often fatal.

Effaced: Shortened.

Embryo: Developmental stage during pregnancy occurring after implantation in the uterus and before about 8 weeks of the pregnancy.

Emergency c-section: Cesarean section performed because the mother or baby is in distress or imminent danger.

Endocrine: Hormone-related.

Estriol: A variant of estrogen that is produced primarily by the placenta during pregnancy.

Estrogen: A female reproductive hormone.

Exit procedure: Surgery on a fetus prior to completing a cesarean section.

F

Fallopian tube: Tube connecting the ovaries to the uterus, through which an egg passes after ovulation.

Fetal alcohol spectrum disorder: A collection of physical effects on the fetus caused by alcohol consumption during pregnancy.

Fetal alcohol syndrome: Significant physical and mental impairment caused by high levels of alcohol consumption during pregnancy.

Fetal fibronectin test: A blood test that measures levels of the "glue" holding the fetus in the uterus to determine whether labor may be imminent.

Fetal nuchal translucency: The translucent space at the back of the fetus's neck.

Fetoscopic surgery: A surgical technique for operating on a fetus while in the uterus using laparoscopic methods.

Fetus: Developmental stage during pregnancy occurring after about 8 weeks of the pregnancy until birth.

First trimester screening: A screening test performed in weeks 11–14 that combines nuchal fold translucency with blood tests to look for chromosome abnormalities in the fetus.

First trimester screening: A combination of blood and urine tests and ultrasound screening to look for early signs of complications in the first trimester.

Fundal height: Measurement of uterine expansion over the course of pregnancy.

G

Gastroschisis: A condition in the fetus in which a hole in the abdominal wall causes part of the intestines to spill out into the amniotic sac.

Genetic mutations: Alterations to DNA that occur randomly.

Gestational diabetes: Diabetes that occurs directly as a result of pregnancy.

Glucose: Blood sugar.

Group B strep: A specific form of streptococcal bacteria.

H

HELLP syndrome: A life-threatening hypertensive disorder of pregnancy characterized by liver dysfunction.

Hemoglobin: A protein in red blood cells that binds oxygen from the lungs and transports it to tissues throughout the body.

Hemolytic disease of the newborn: A condition in which the mother's immune system attacks the fetus because of different Rh factors in their blood.

Hormones: Chemicals produced by various organs to produce specific responses by body systems.

Hospitalized bed rest: Complete bed rest that takes place in a hospital.

Human chorionic gonadotrophin (hCG): A hormone produced by the placenta that prevents menstruation and ovulation.

Human placental lactogen (HPL): A hormone produced by the placenta that interferes with insulin to promote growth in the fetus.

Hyperemesis gravidarum: Excessive vomiting during pregnancy.

Hypertension: High blood pressure.

I

Immune suppression: Treatment to decrease immune system activity.

Incompetent cervix: A cervix that is weak or thin and therefore opens prematurely during pregnancy.

Induced: Caused to occur artificially.

Inherited disorder: An illness or disorder caused by defects in genes passed to the child by one or both parents.

Insulin: A hormone produced by the pancreas that processes glucose.

Insulin resistance: A condition in which the body does not respond properly to insulin in the bloodstream.

Intrahepatic cholestasis of pregnancy (ICP): A liver disorder in which bile doesn't flow properly through ducts in the liver, causing itchy skin and potentially life-threatening complications.

Intrauterine growth restriction (IUGR): A condition in which a fetus does not grow at the rate normally expected.

Iron-deficiency anemia: A condition in which a person has too little iron in his or her blood for hemoglobin to transport oxygen effectively.

J

Jaundice: Yellowing of the skin.

K

Karyotyping: Chromosome analysis.

L

Leukemia: Any of several forms of cancer affecting the white blood cells.

Leukorrhea: Milky vaginal discharge.

Listeriosis: A bacterial infection found in raw or undercooked meats.

M

Maternal/fetal medicine specialist: A physician specializing in treatment of high-risk pregnancies.

Maternal serum alpha-fetoprotein (MSAFP): A blood test measuring levels of alpha-fetoprotein to assess the risk of certain birth defects.

Meconium aspiration: Inhalation of stools passed in utero.

Modified bed rest: Bed rest in which the mother may get up periodically but should stay in bed most of the time.

N

Nausea and vomiting of pregnancy: A symptom of pregnancy commonly occurring in the first trimester.

Necrotizing enterocolitis: A gastrointestinal disease, usually affecting premature infants, in which infection and inflammation damage the intestine.

Neonatal intensive care unit (NICU): A specialized facility in a hospital where ill or premature babies are cared for.

Neural tube defects: Birth defects affecting the development of the spine and/or brain.

Newborn/Neonate: A newly born infant; a baby less than a month old.

Nondisjunction: Abnormal division of a fertilized egg resulting in missing or extra chromosomes.

Nuchal cord: Umbilical cord wrapped around the neck of the fetus.

Nuchal translucency scan: An ultrasound analysis in the first trimester used to assess the risk of certain congenital disorders, especially Down syndrome.

Nucleus: The structure within a cell that contains the cell's genetic matter.

O

Oligohydramnios: Low amniotic fluid.

Open fetal surgery: A surgical technique for operating on a fetus that involves opening up the uterus, performing surgery, and restoring the fetus to the uterus.

Oral glucose tolerance test: A test to determine how a pregnant woman's body responds to glucose; a gestational diabetes test.

Ovaries: Reproductive organs in women where eggs (ova) are stored and certain hormones are released.

Ovulates: The release of an egg in the ovaries midway through a woman's reproductive cycle.

Ovum: Egg.

Oxytocin: A hormone and neurotransmitter that is important in labor.

P

Perinatologist: *See maternal/fetal specialist.*

Pica: Cravings for dirt, ice, or other nonnutritive substances while pregnant.

Placenta: Specialized organ that develops to supply oxygen and nutrients to a growing fetus.

Placenta previa: A condition in which the placenta partially or completely covers the cervix.

Placental abruption: A condition in which the placenta has pulled away from the wall of the uterus prior to birth.

Polycythemia: Excess red blood cells.

Population studies: Research that examines large groups of people to determine what proportion of the population may experience certain phenomena.

Predispose: Having an increased risk.

Preeclampsia: A hypertensive disorder of pregnancy.

Pregnancy-induced hypertension: Elevated blood pressure caused by pregnancy.

Prenatal testing: A collection of diagnostic tests that can suggest or confirm disorders in the fetus.

Prenatal vitamin: A vitamin formulated to suit the needs of pregnant women.

Preterm labor: Labor that begins prior to the 37th week of pregnancy.

Probability: A measurement of the likelihood of an event actually occurring.

Progesterone: A female hormone with several important roles in pregnancy.

Prolactin: A hormone that is associated with milk production.

Prostaglandin: A hormone-like substance important in the contraction and relaxation of smooth muscle, the dilation and constriction of blood vessels, control of blood pressure, and modulation of inflammation.

Pruritic urticarial papules and plaques of pregnancy (PUPPP): An itchy rash that occurs in pregnancy for unknown reasons.

Pulmonary function testing: Testing to determine how well lungs transfer oxygen into the bloodstream.

Pulmonologist: A doctor specializing in lung disease.

Q

Quad screen: Screening for levels of four key hormones—MSAFP, hCG, estriol, and inhibin—that if abnormal can suggest potential problems with a pregnancy.

R

Relaxin: A hormone that causes loosening of ligaments and cervical ripening prior to labor.

Remission: Temporary cessation of disease.

Respiratory distress syndrome (RDS): Poor lung function in premature infants that is often caused by lack of surfactant in the lungs.

Rh status: The presence or absence of a specific blood factor that can determine the risk of hemolytic disease of the newborn.

Risk: A determination of the probability of a particular event that takes into account specific contributing factors.

S

Screening tests: Diagnostic tools used to assess a risk of specific disorders in pregnancy.

Second trimester screening: A series of tests, including ultrasound and the "quad screen" used to determine the risk of birth defects, especially neural tube defects.

Sexually transmitted disease (STD): Any of several diseases passed between sexual partners.

Small for gestational age (SGA): *See intrauterine growth restriction.*

Sperm: Male reproductive cell that joins with an ovum to initiate pregnancy.

Statistic: A numerical summation of data collected during research.

Stillbirth: Death of the fetus after the 20th week of pregnancy.

Strict bed rest: Confinement to bed except for use of the bathroom.

Sudden infant death syndrome (SIDS): Unexplained sudden death of a newborn or very young child.

Surfactant: A substance in the lungs that enables lung tissue to move more easily.

Systolic: Blood pressure during the exertion phase of the heartbeat.

T

Thrombocytopenia: Low platelet count.

Thrombophilias: Factors that cause blood to clot more readily.

Thyroxine: A hormone produced by the thyroid gland.

Tocolytic medications: Medications that can temporarily halt premature contractions.

Torsions: Umbilical cord twisted around a limb or knotted around itself.

Toxemia: *See preeclampsia.*

Toxoplasmosis: A bacterial infection carried in raw meat and occasionally found in cats.

Twin transfusion syndrome: A condition in which identical twins that share a placenta have unequal amounts of blood in their bodies.

Type 1 diabetes: Diabetes occurring because insulin is not produced by the pancreas.

Type 2 diabetes: Diabetes occurring either because the pancreas decreases its production of insulin, or the body has developed insulin resistance.

U

Ultrasound bonding: An emotional bond created between parents and the fetus when the fetus is viewed by ultrasound.

Ultrasound fetal survey: An ultrasound examination of the physical status and position of the fetus, umbilical cord, and placenta.

Ultrasound specialist: A medical professional trained in the use of ultrasound scanning to assess and diagnose pregnancy and pregnancy-related disorders.

Umbilical cord: The cord connecting the placenta to the fetus.

Uterus: Female reproductive organ used for carrying the fetus during pregnancy.

V

Vasoconstrictor: Causing narrowing of the blood vessels.

Index

Index

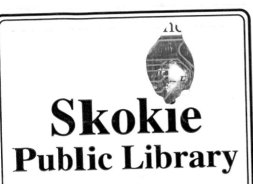

www.jbpub.com

100 QUESTIONS & ANSWERS

Elizabeth S. Platt
Michael G. Pinette, MD
Betty Campbell, RN
Andrea Tetreau, RN

About Your High-Risk Pregnancy

EMPOWER YOURSELF !

100 Questions & Answers About Your High-Risk Pregnancy provides authoritative, practical answers to the most common questions posed by "at-risk" expecting mothers and fathers. The text covers topics such as testing, mother's health, fetal health, complications, prevention and treatment, and physical and psychological coping. This book is an invaluable resource for anyone coping with the physical and emotional turmoil of high-risk pregnancy.

Questions include:
What happens during a normal pregnancy?
What problems can occur in pregnancy?
Why does my doctor think that I may be at risk?

"*100 Questions & Answers About Your High-Risk Pregnancy* offers an exceptionally comprehensive and thoughtful examination of high-risk pregnancies. It provides medical expertise in a tone that is both accessible and supportive, balancing technical details with personal anecdotes and addressing difficult topics with grace and compassion. As a high-risk patient myself, I felt comforted by the authors' sensitivity and buoyed by their encouragement."

— **Amy O'Keefe**, patient

Jones and Bartlett Publishers
40 Tall Pine Drive
Sudbury, MA 01776
978-443-5000
info@jbpub.com
www.jbpub.com

ISBN13   978-0-7637-5573-7
ISBN10   0-7637-5573-7